MRI Training Console
Lab Book
S version

First Edition

Ken Meacham, PhD (RT)(R)(CT)(MR), CIIP
The Institute for Advanced Clinical Imaging

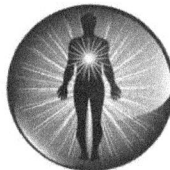

THE INSTITUTE FOR
ADVANCED CLINICAL IMAGING

 www.iacionline.com

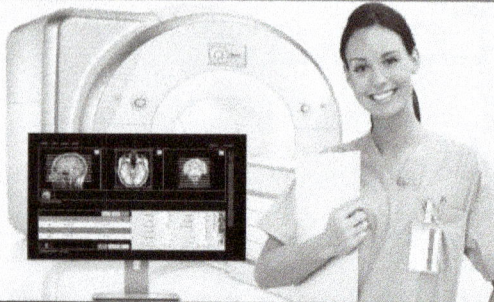

Introducing the
MRI Training Console S

The MRI Training Console allows for the clinical instruction of MRI procedures within the classroom. Students will acquire clinical experience and confidence with the life-like MRI operator's console.

Students will gain knowledge of:

- Coil selection
- Scanning procedures
- Protocol setup
- Sequence selection
- Anatomical coverage
- Parameters and tradeoffs
- Image weighting and Contrast

Instructors can track student progress and make adjustments to parameters in order to improve the student's learning experience.

For more information and a free demo:
www.iacionline.com/simulators.da

THE INSTITUTE FOR
ADVANCED CLINICAL IMAGING

The MRI Training Console Software

The MRI Simulator software was designed to provide clinical hands-on training to students within the classroom. While we have worked to make this product as life-like as possible, some functions are too complex to simulate. However, we do believe we have developed an outstanding learning tool. For more information and to demo this product visit: **www.iacionline.com/simulators.da.**

The MRI Training Console Lab Book

This lab book was designed as a companion to the MRI simulator software developed by The Institute for advanced clinical imaging (IACI) . These products were developed in direct response to feedback provided by the MRI and CT students of IACI. I am extremely grateful to all of the students whose feedback has been invaluable to the improvement of our programs. For more information about the programs at IACI visit: **www.iacionline.com.**

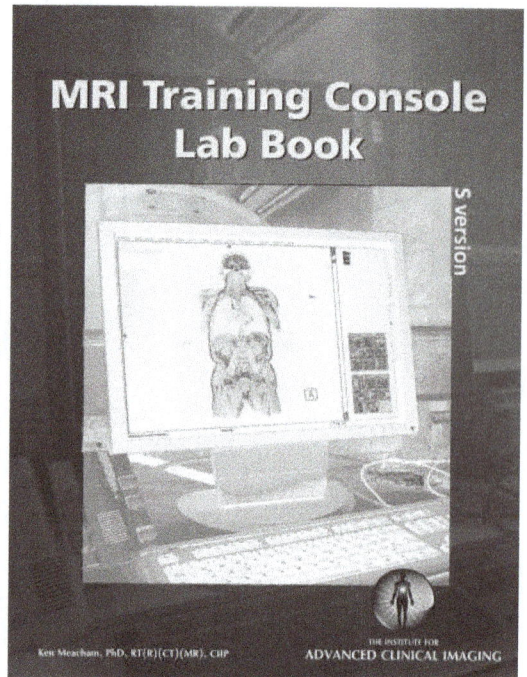

MRI Training Console Lab Book
S version

Ken Meacham, PhD, RT(R)(CT)(MR), CHP

THE INSTITUTE FOR
ADVANCED CLINICAL IMAGING

The Institute for Advanced Clinical Imaging
5261 Highland Road, Suite 170
Baton Rouge, LA 70808
www.iacionline.com
Email: info@iacionline.net

Table of Contents

Navigate the MRI Training Console

Objective:

In this lab you will learn to navigate features and options associated with the MRI training consul

Step - By—Step

1. Before using the MRI training consul, your instructor should have created a user account for you.

2. take a moment to review the buttons and settings on the primary MRI scanning console.

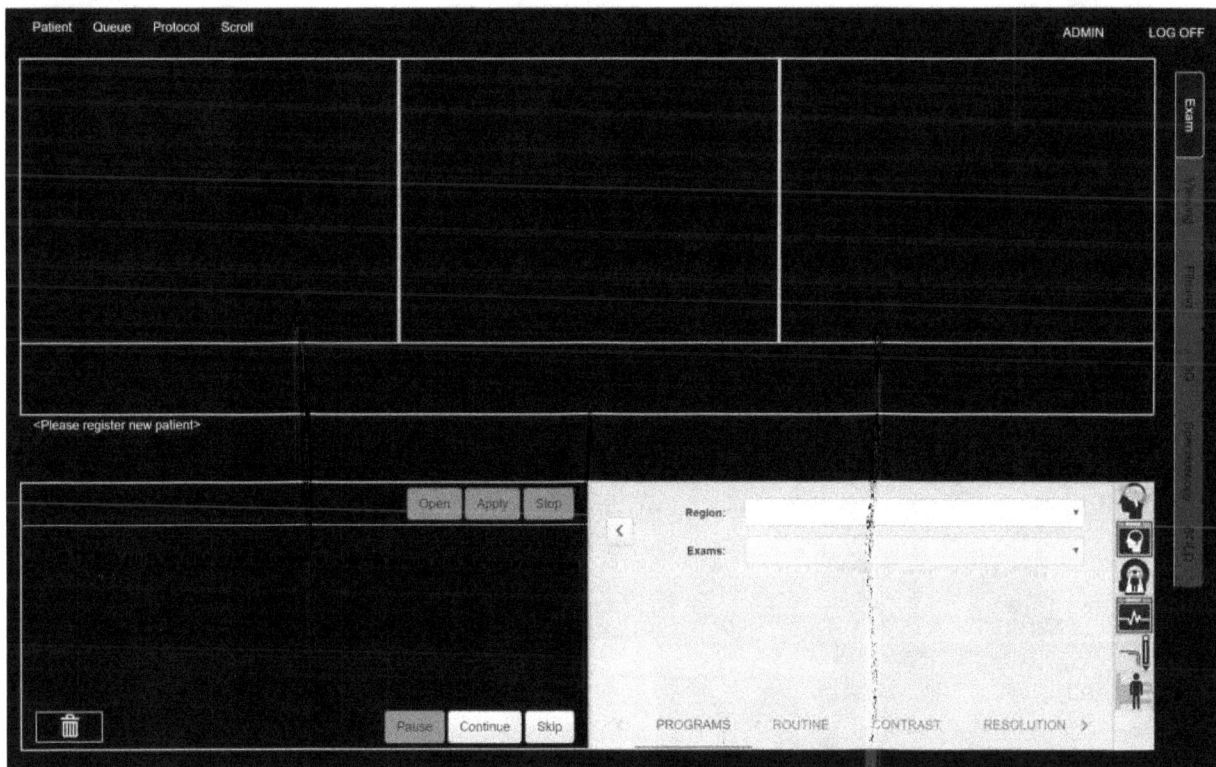

3. Menu—The menu area is used to register the patient and control scan options during the use of the simulator.

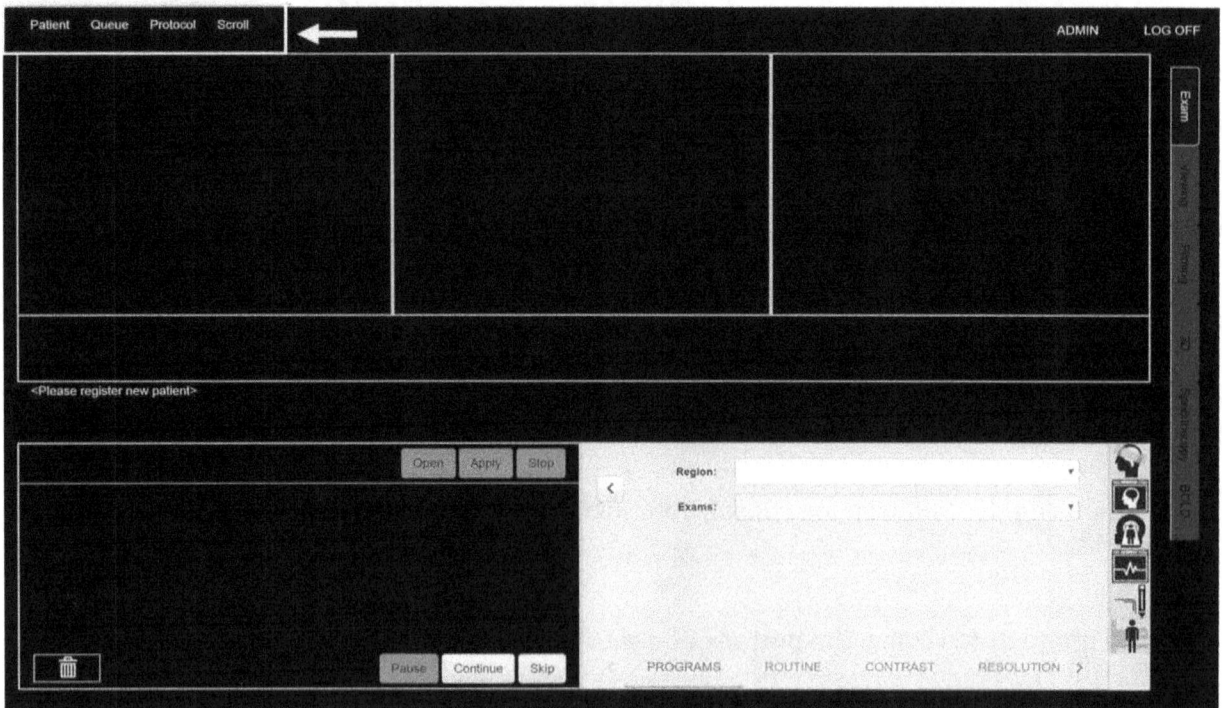

4. Patient Menu— The patient menu allows the student to register the patient and end the exam.

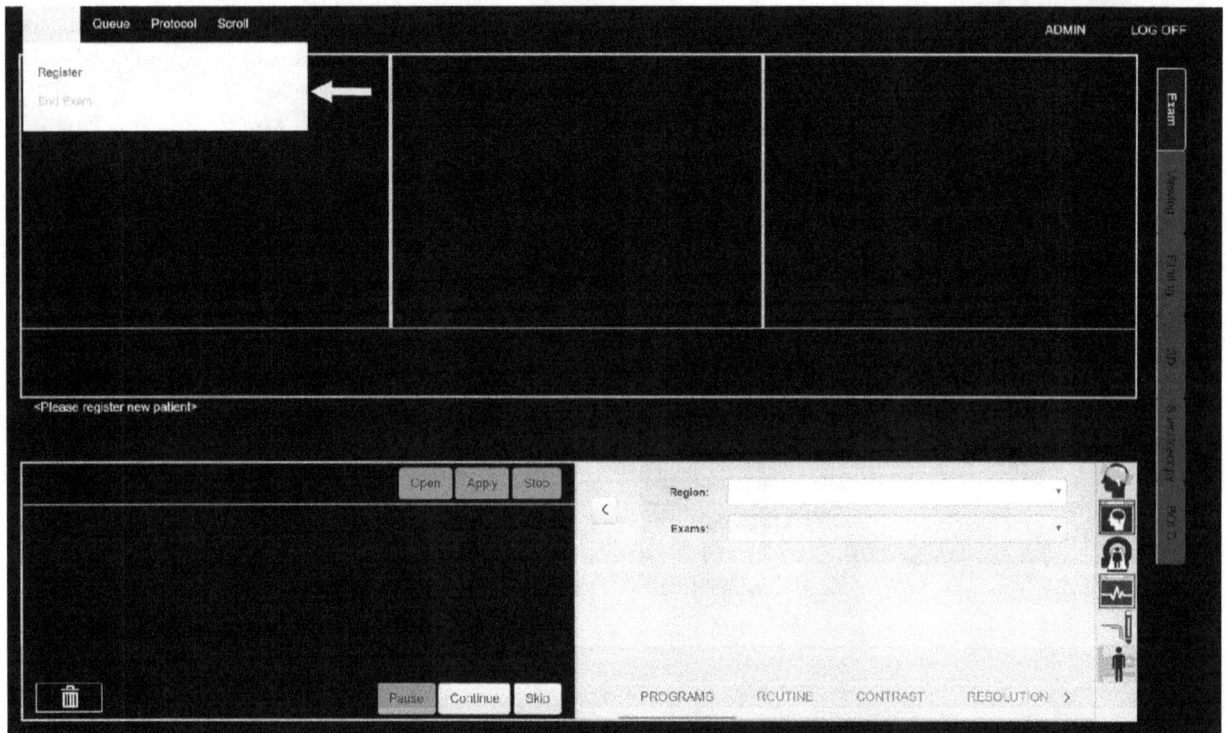

5. Queue menu— The queue menu allows the user to control the active sequence, select the coil, and document the use of contrast.

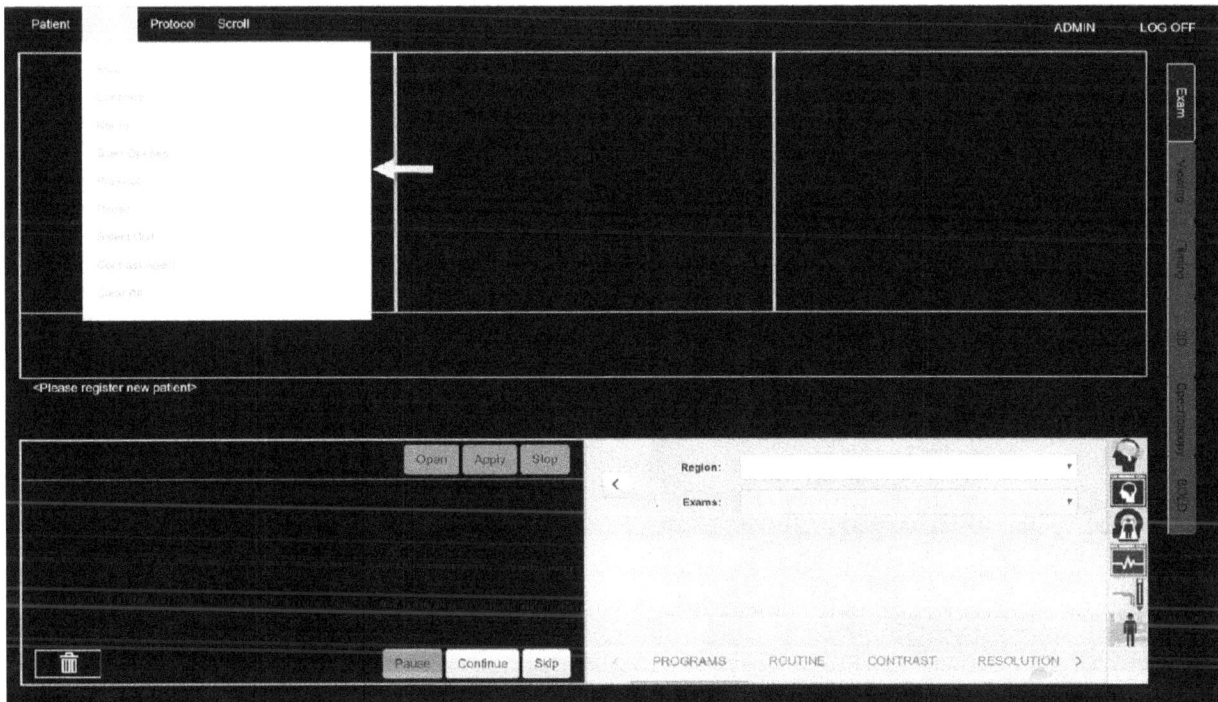

6. Protocol menu—The protocol menu allows the user to plan the sequence slices and saturation pulses.

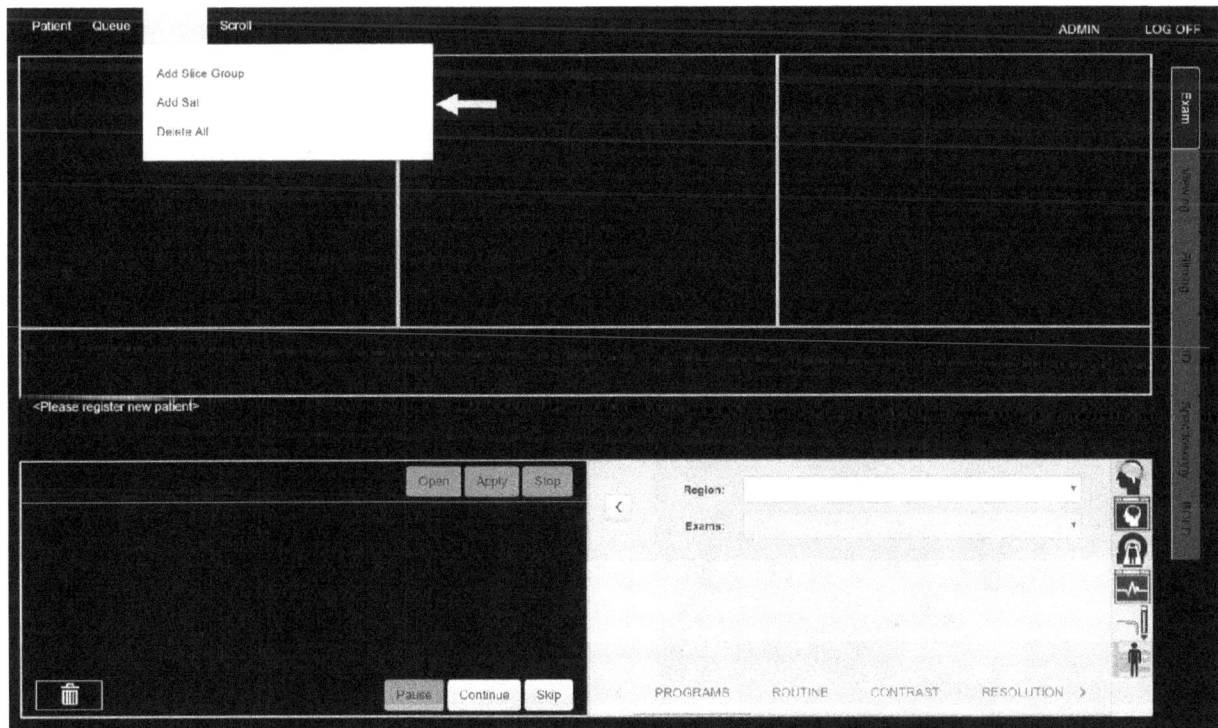

7. Scroll Menu— The scroll menu allows the users to navigate images and sequences.

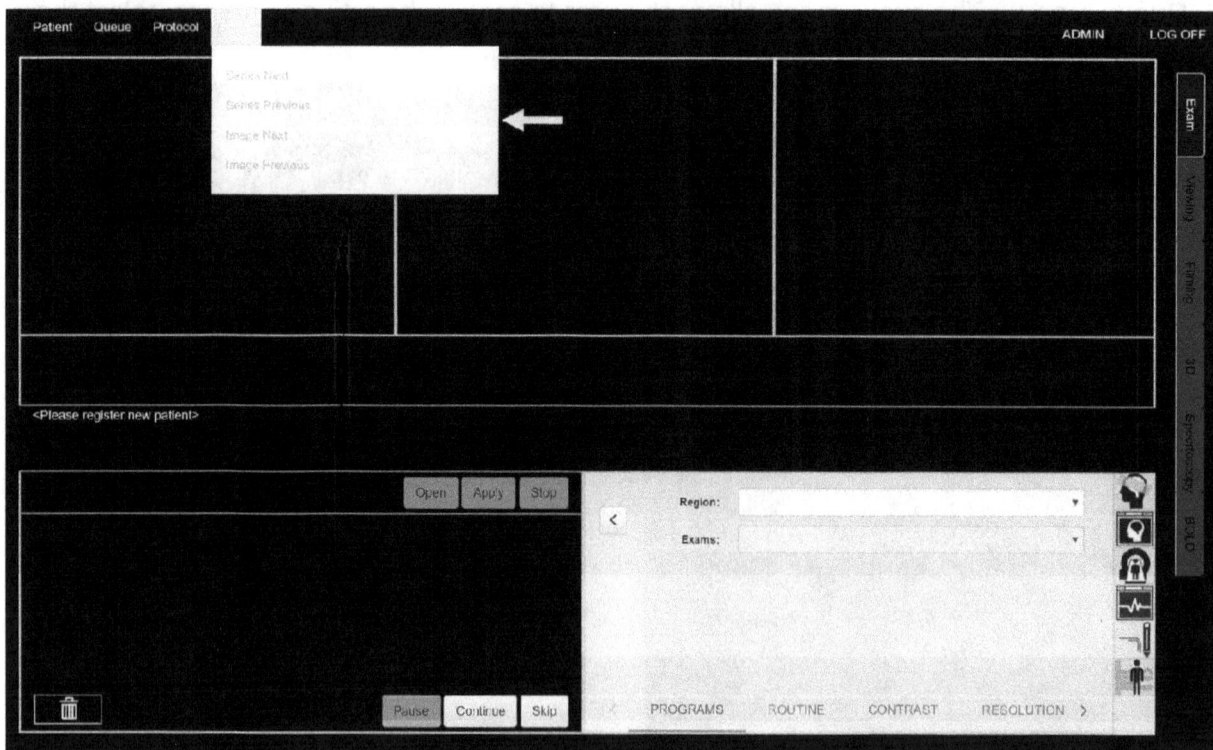

8. Admin/Logoff—The admin area allows the instructor to manage the user accounts and laboratory parameters. The logoff button will log the user out of the simulator software.

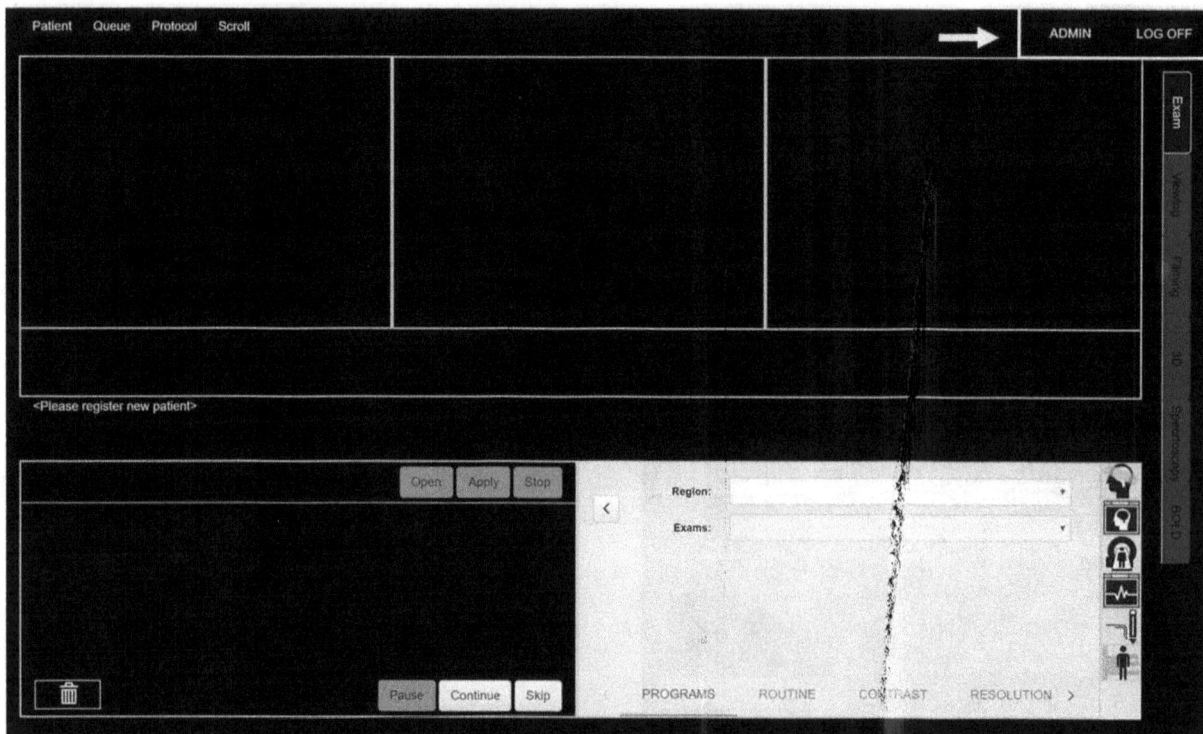

9. Exam Tab—These buttons are inactive and simulate other functions found on an MRI scanner. However, they are not necessary part of learning to scan.

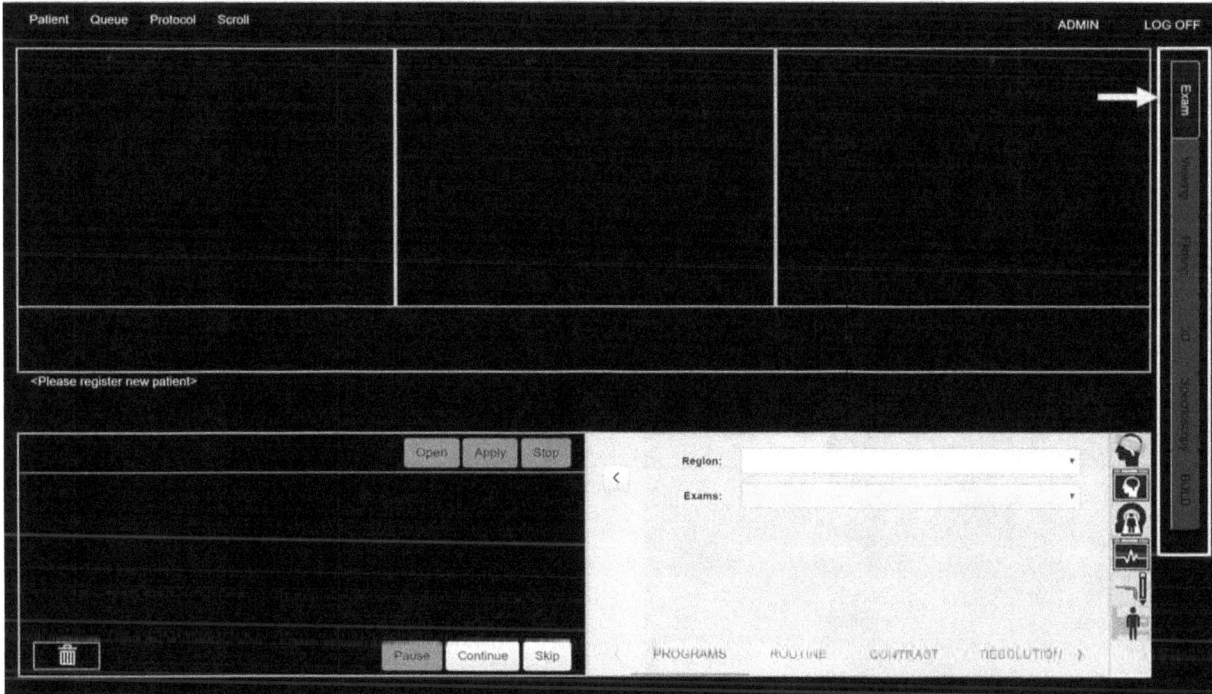

10. Image viewports— The image viewport area displays the images after they are scanned and allows the user to navigate the images and sequences. This area also allows the user to prescribe the slices for each sequence.

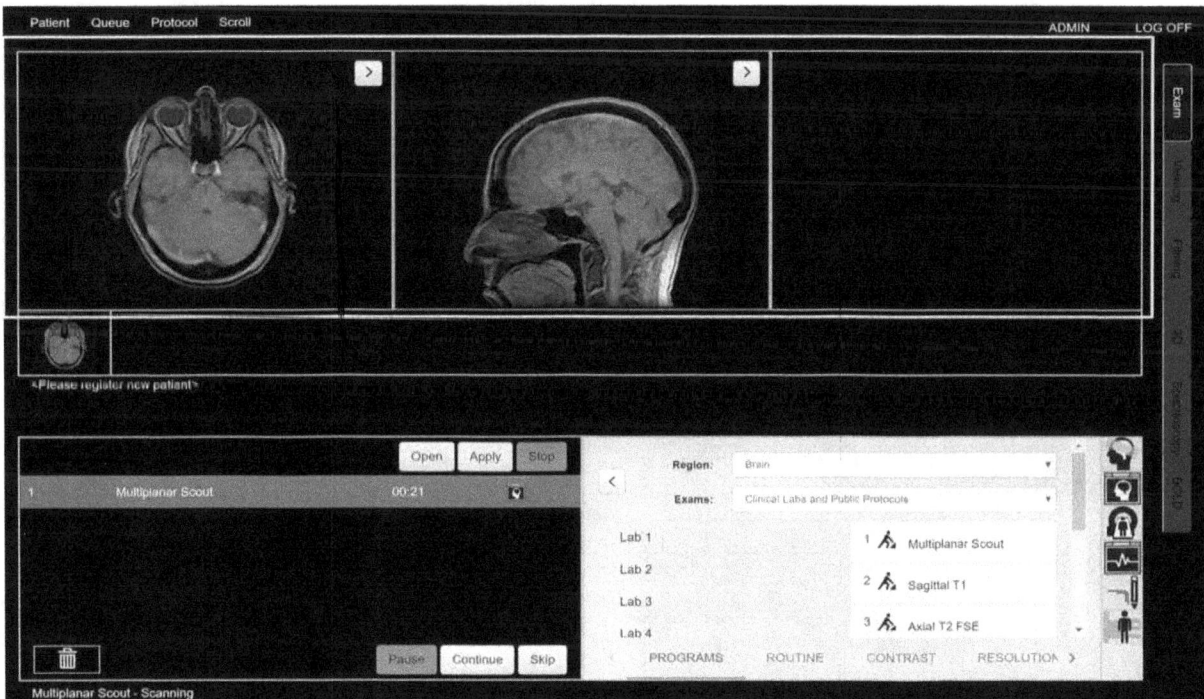

11. Sequence thumbnails—The sequence thumbnail area displays a thumbnail of each sequence scanned. Sequence thumbnails can be dragged and dropped into the viewport area.

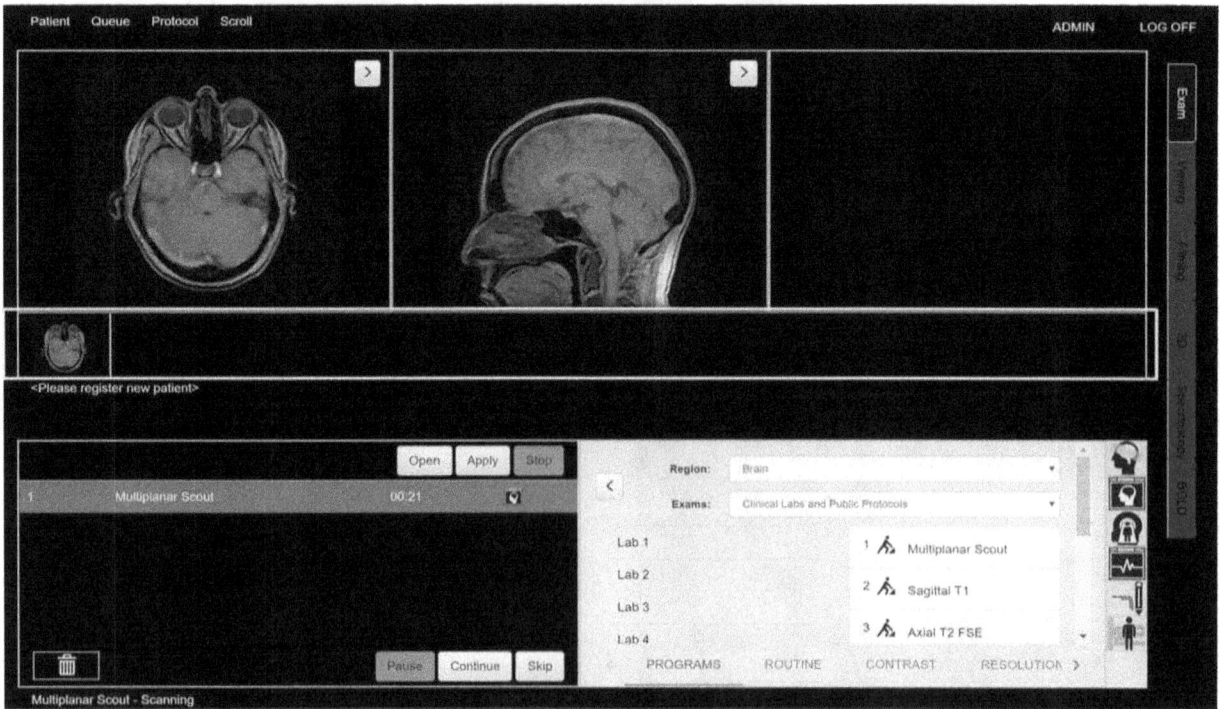

12. Scanning Toolbar—The scanning toolbar provides a series of tools to set up and review the sequences to be scanned.

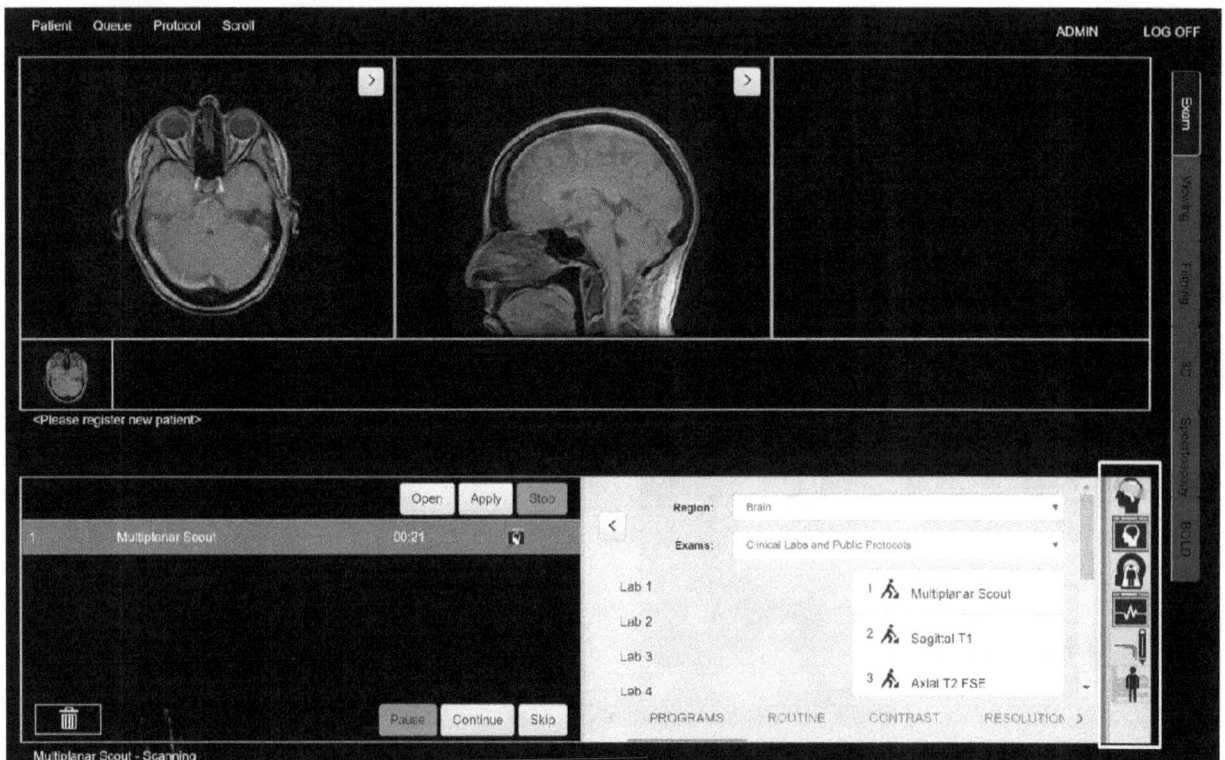

13. Position toolbar— The position toolbar allows users to setup and manipulate sequences as well as MIP reconstructions. Buttons blue in color are active. Grey buttons are inactive.

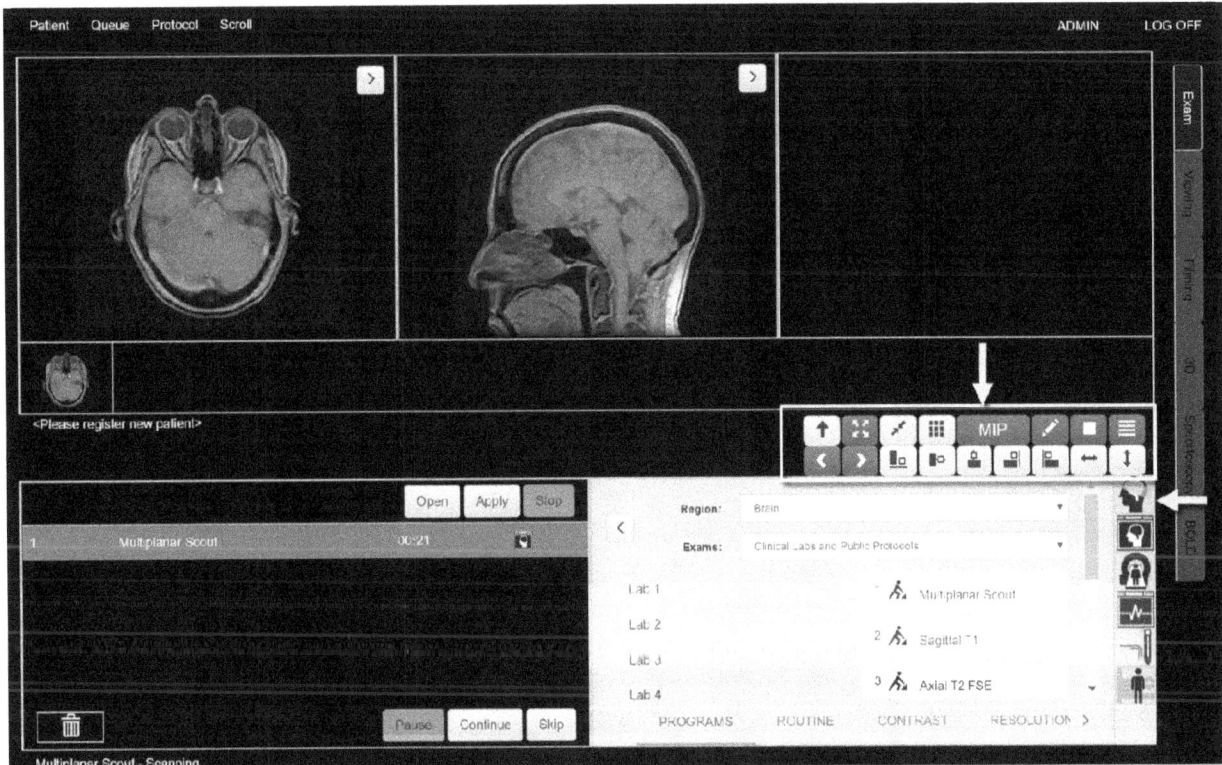

14. Inline display—The inline display button displays the last sequence scanned.

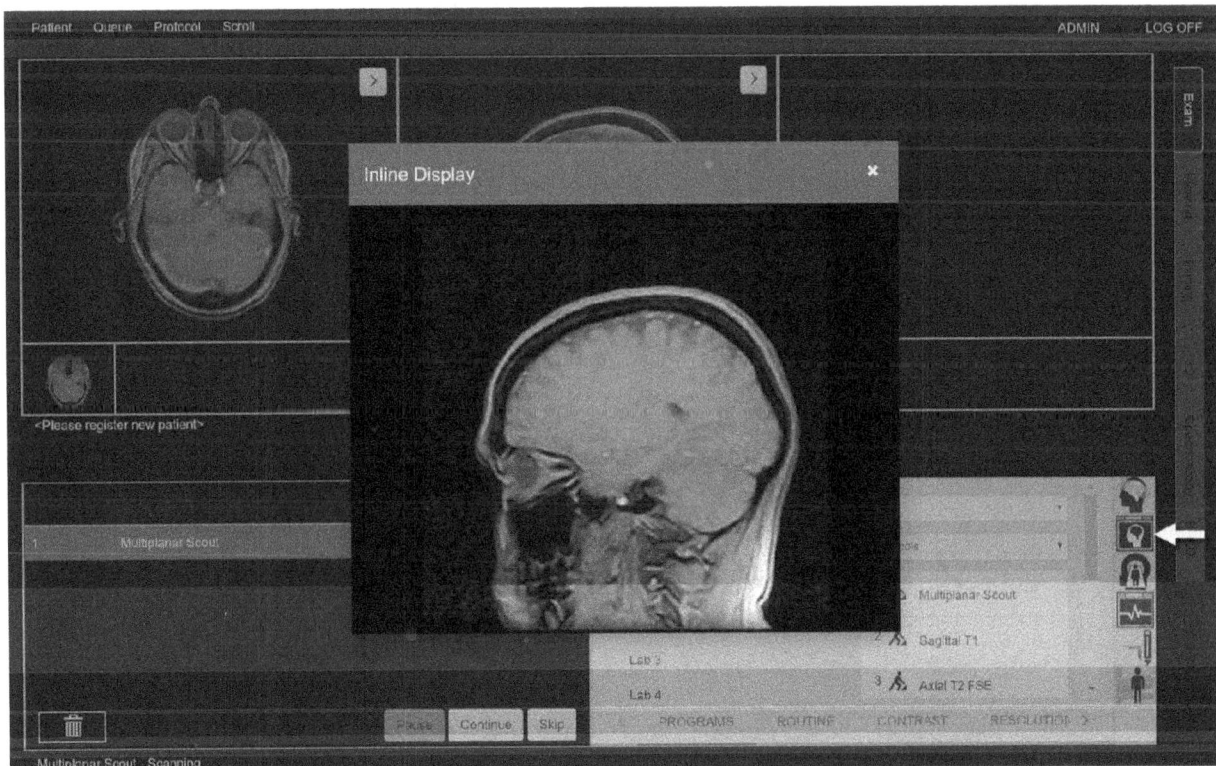

15. Table position—The table position button displays the simulated table position.

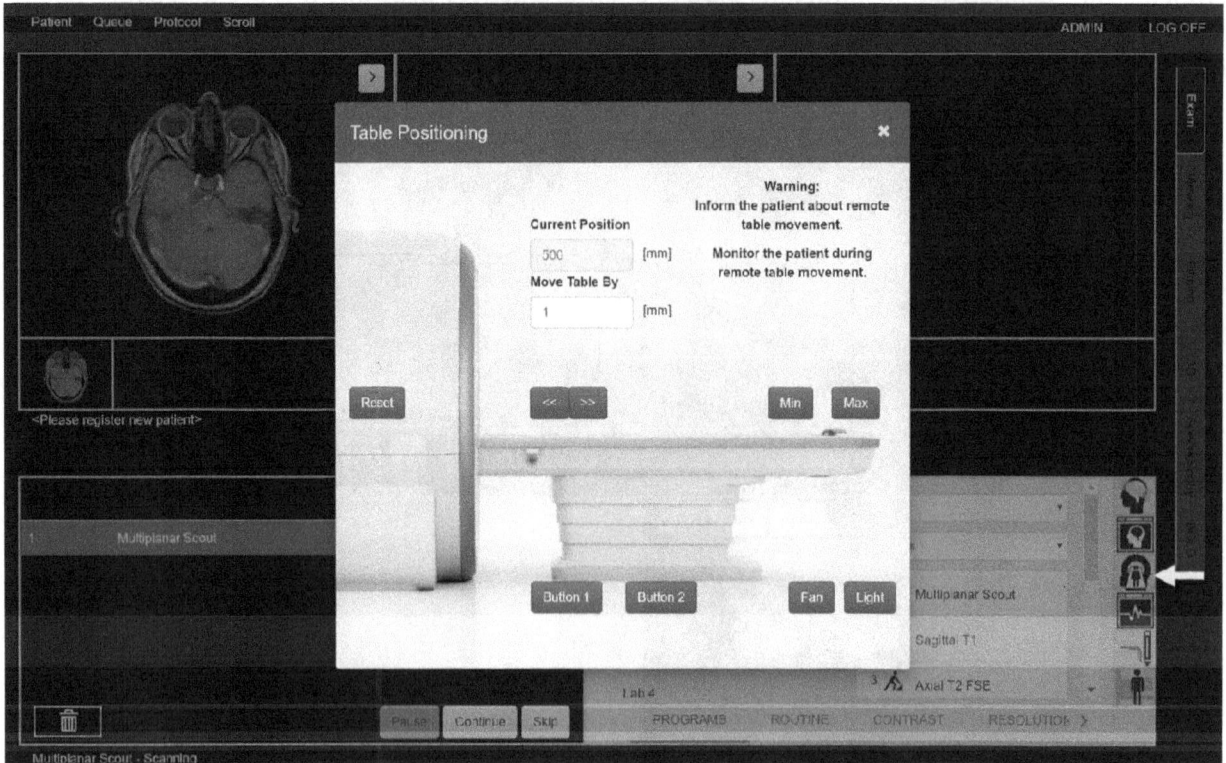

16. Physiological display—The physiological display button displays a the heart rate of the simulated patient.

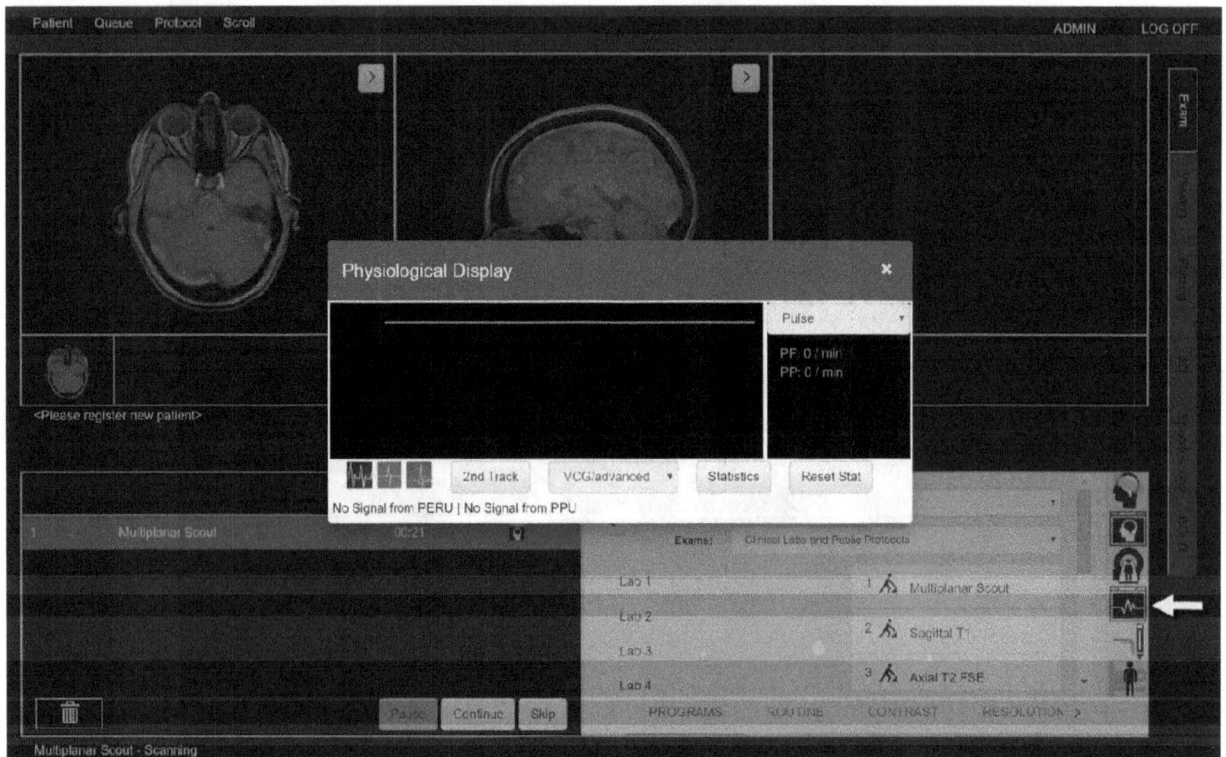

17. Exam explorer The exam explorer allows the user to view and select sequences from the library of protocols.

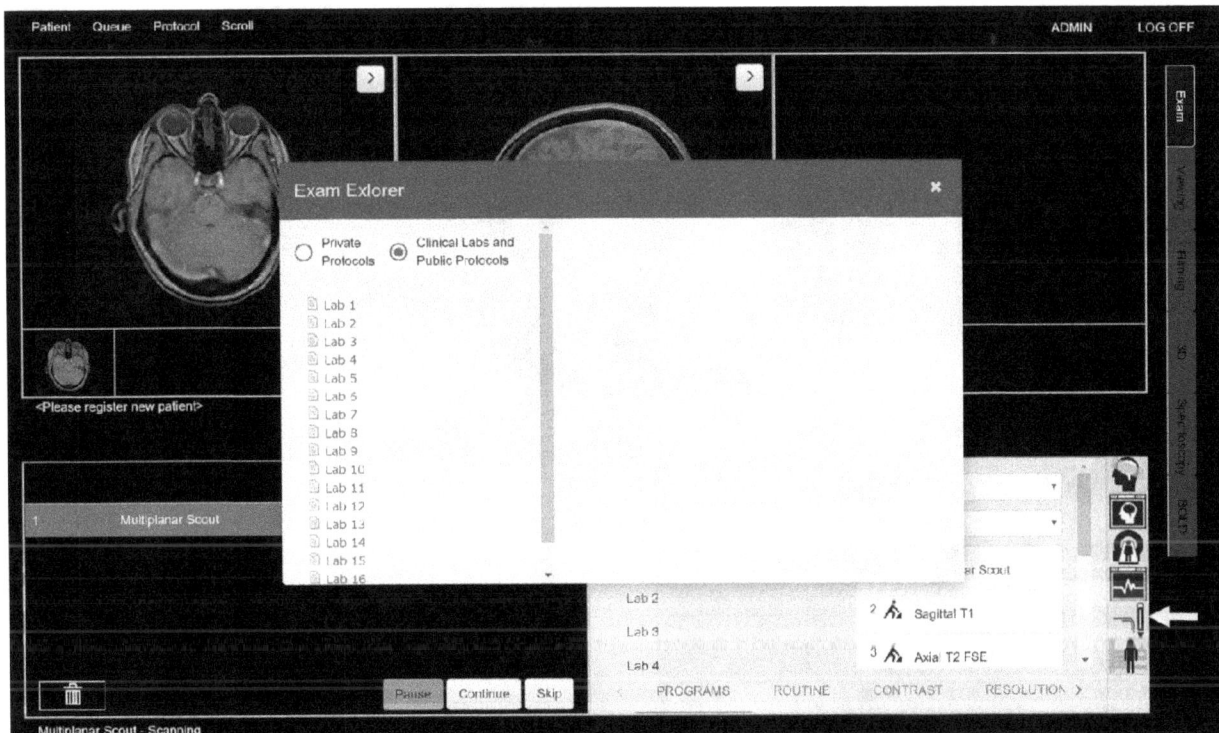

18. SAR information— The SAR information button displays simulated specific absorption rate values.

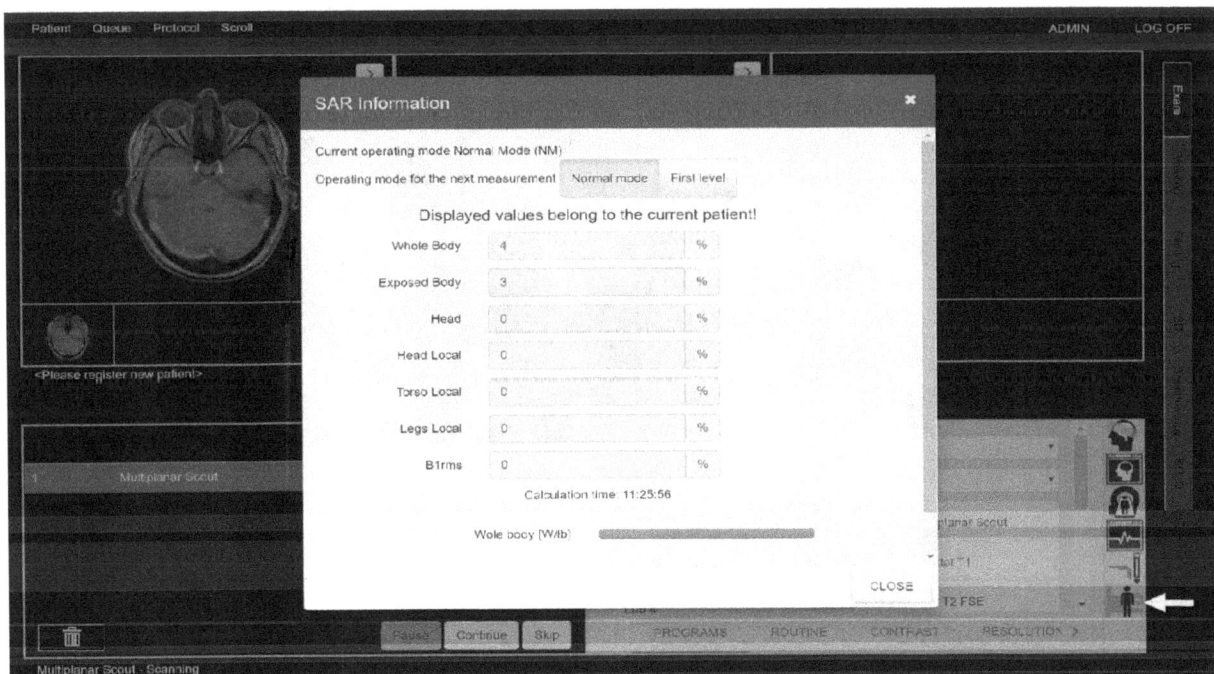

19. Protocol selector—The protocol selector area allows the user to select the protocol and sequences to be scanned. This area also allows the user to edit the sequence parameters.

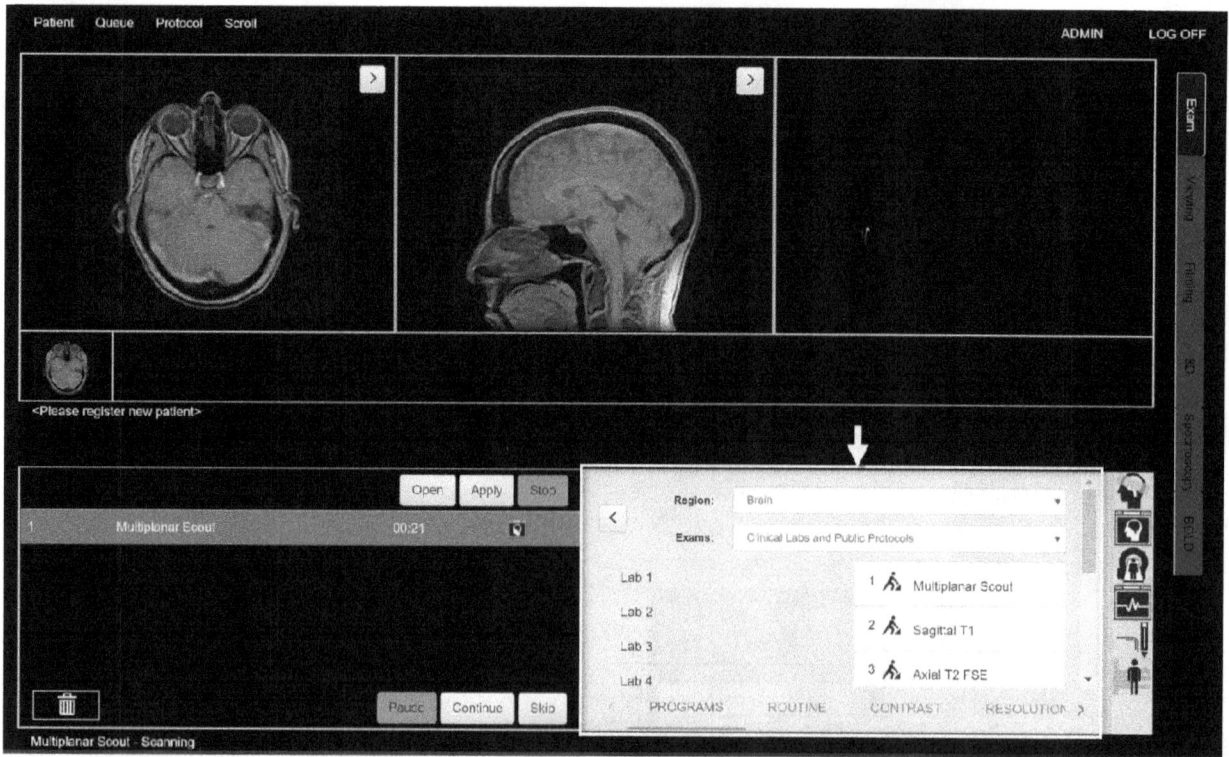

20. Scan manager— The scan manager area allows the user to open, scan, pause, and stop the selected sequences.

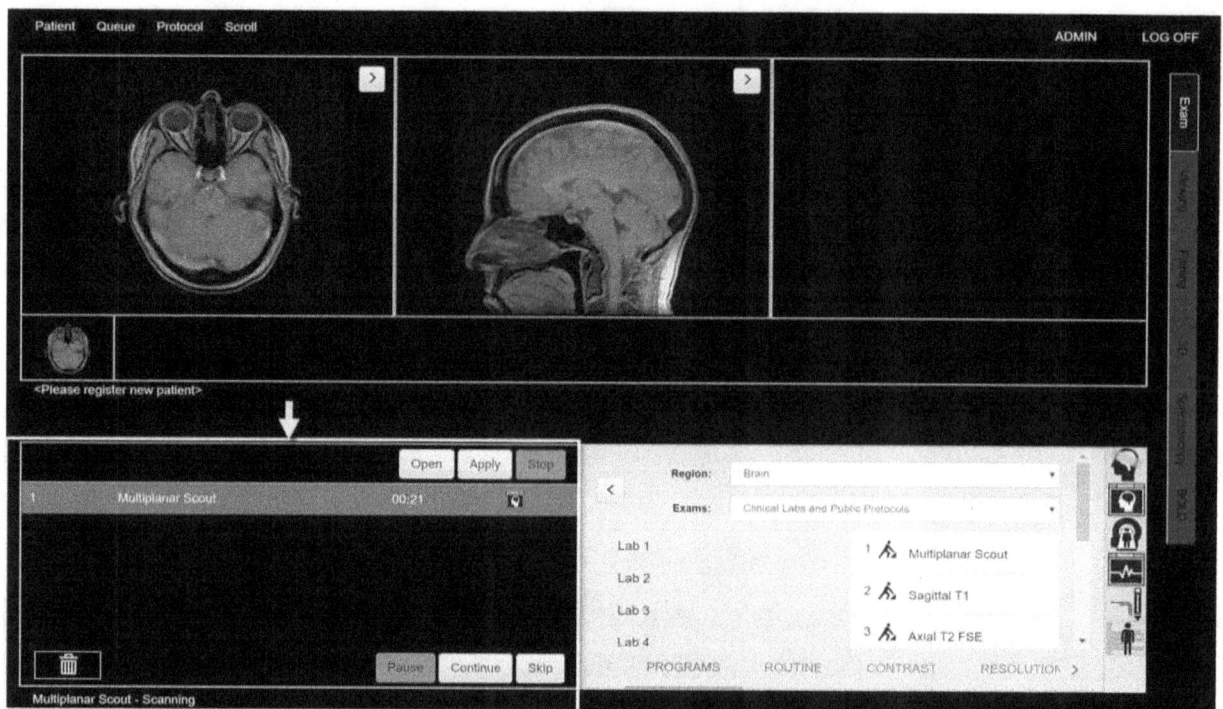

21. Patient Registration—Select patient from the top menu and click the register option. Enter the patient information and click the exam button to register the patient.

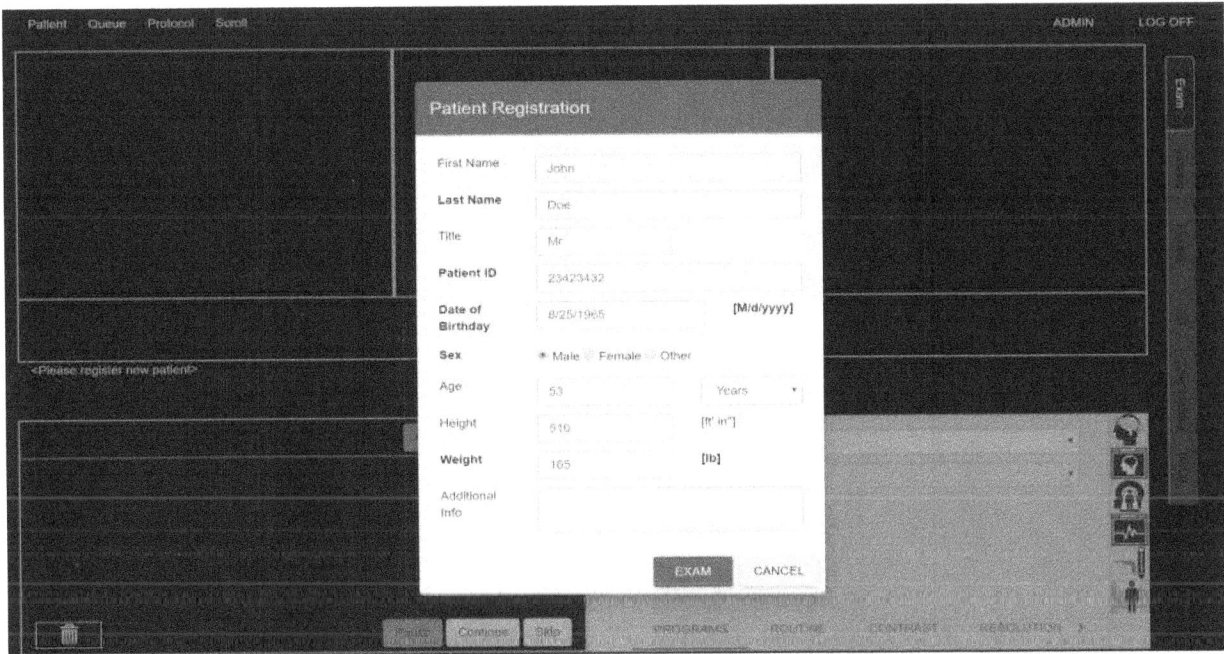

22. Registration Confirmation & Coil Selection— Review the patient information and select the patient orientation. Click the confirm button to confirm the data is correct. Select the Head/Neck coil from the coil options and click the select button to select the coil.

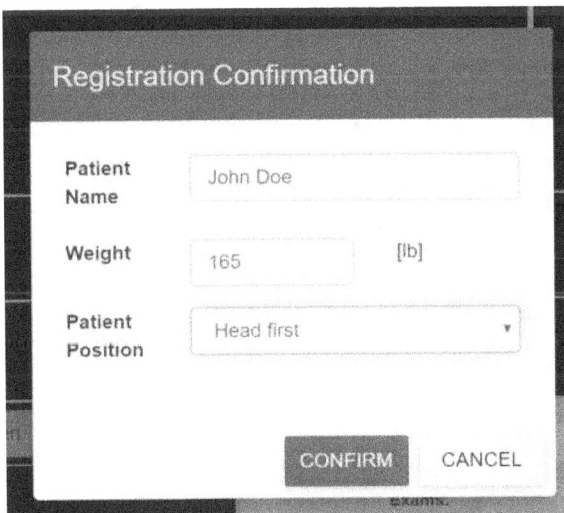

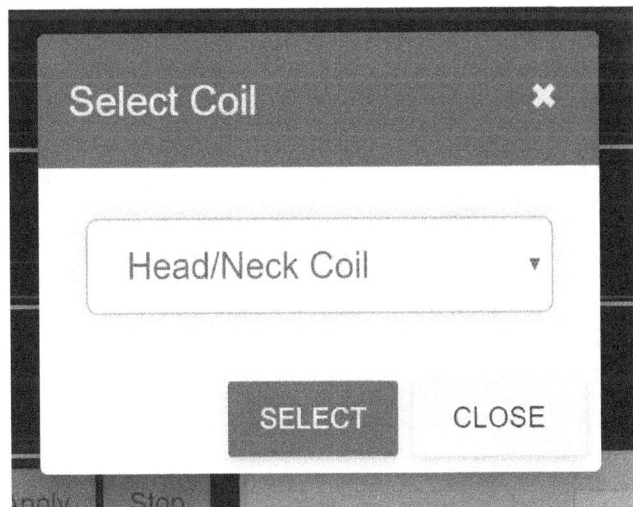

23. Select the protocol—Click the region drop down list and select brain from the list. Select clinical labs and public protocols form the exams dropdown list. Click on Lab 1 to view the sequences within the protocol.

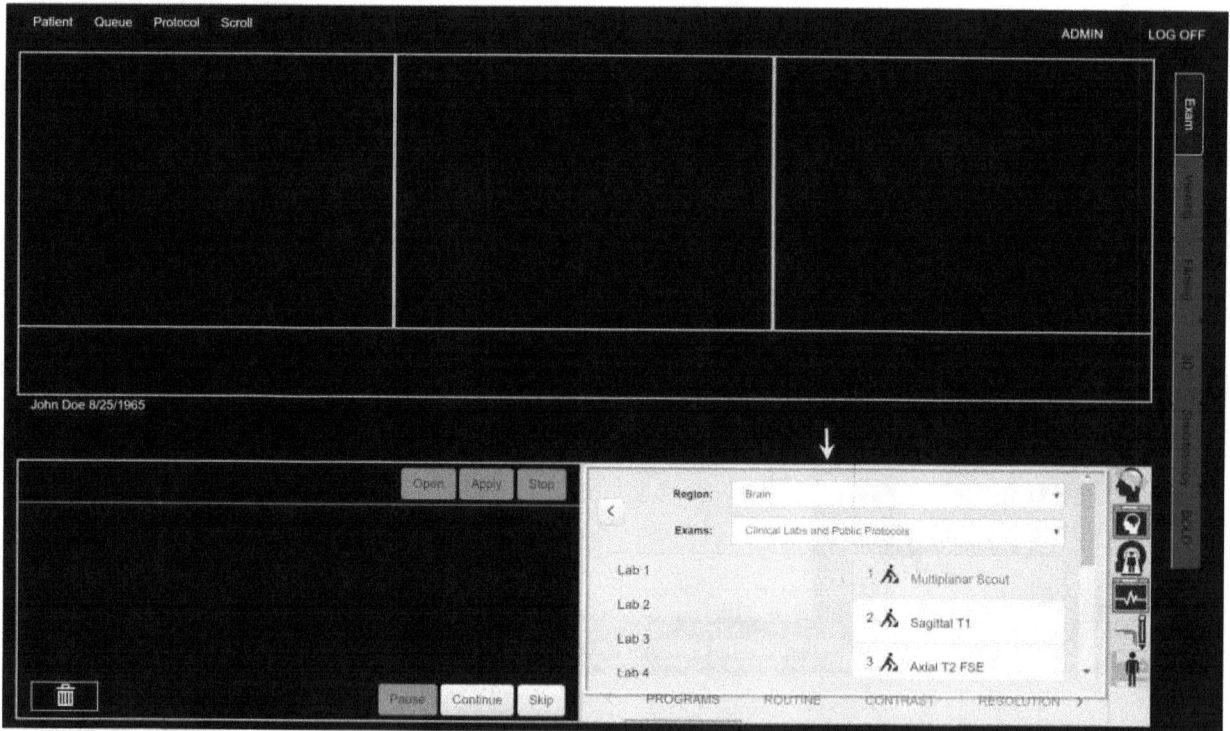

24. Left click on the sequences and drag and drop sequence 1, 2 and 3 to the scan manager area.

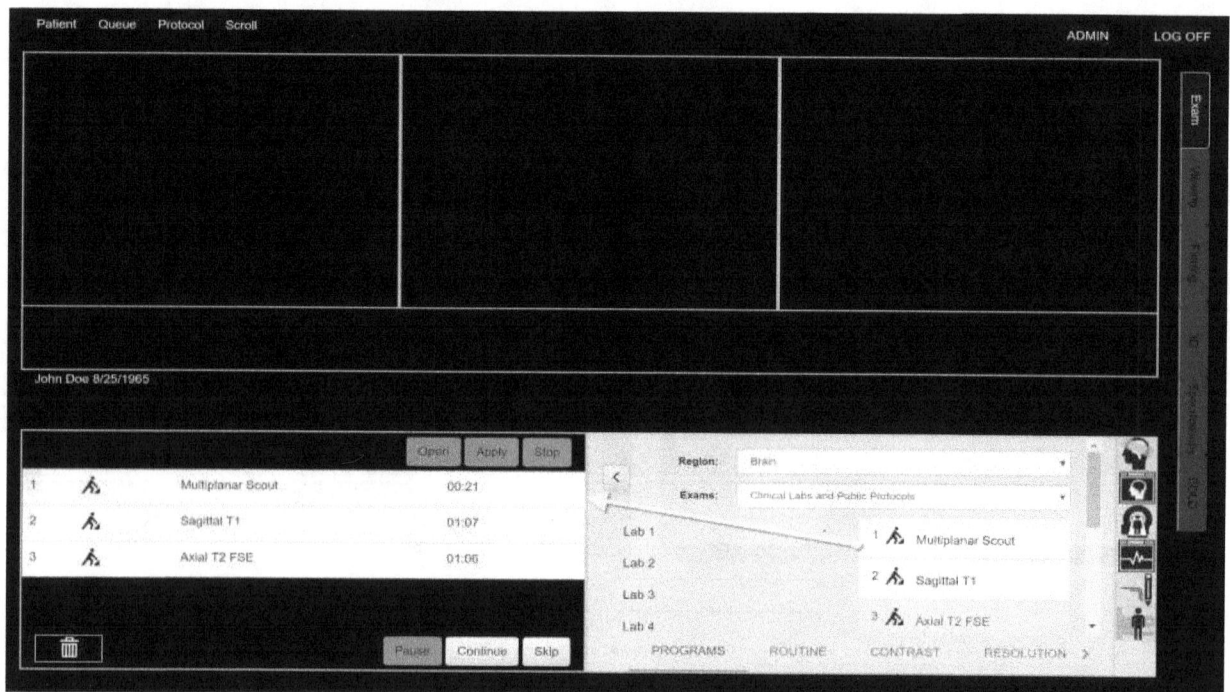

26. Review Sequence Parameters— Select on the first sequence in the scan manager area and click the open button to review the parameters.

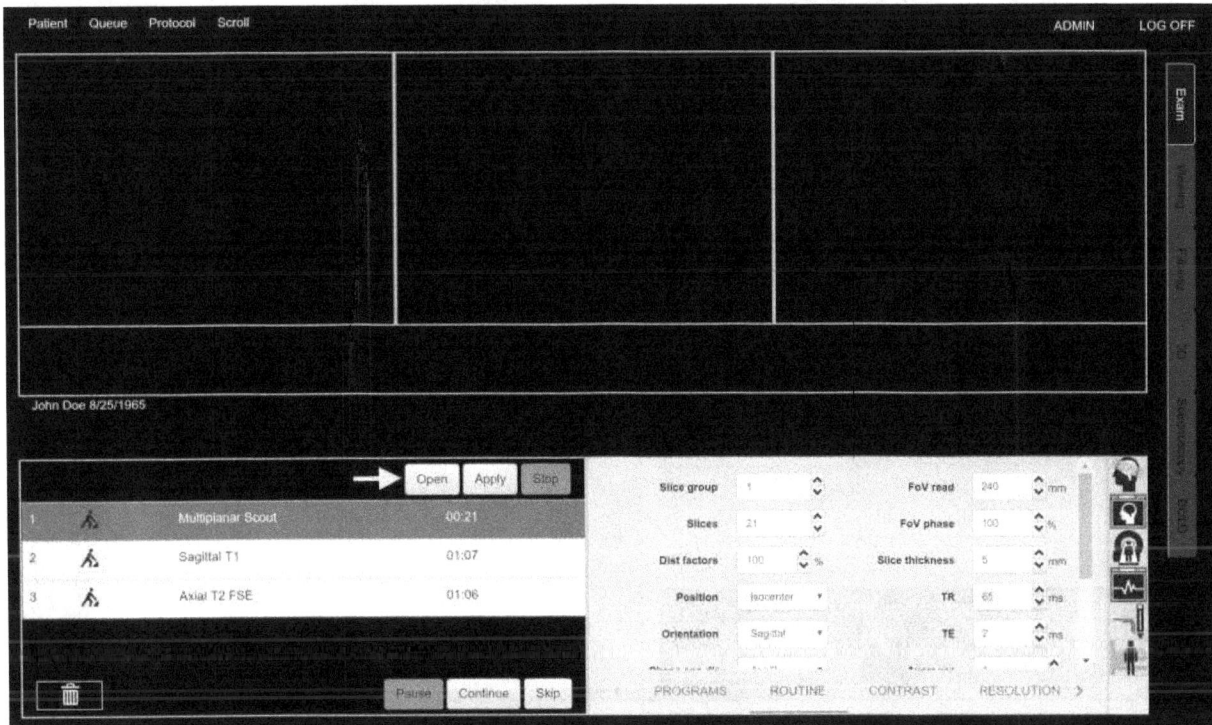

27. Review Sequence Parameters— Select a tab in the parameter area to review the sequence parameters for that tab.

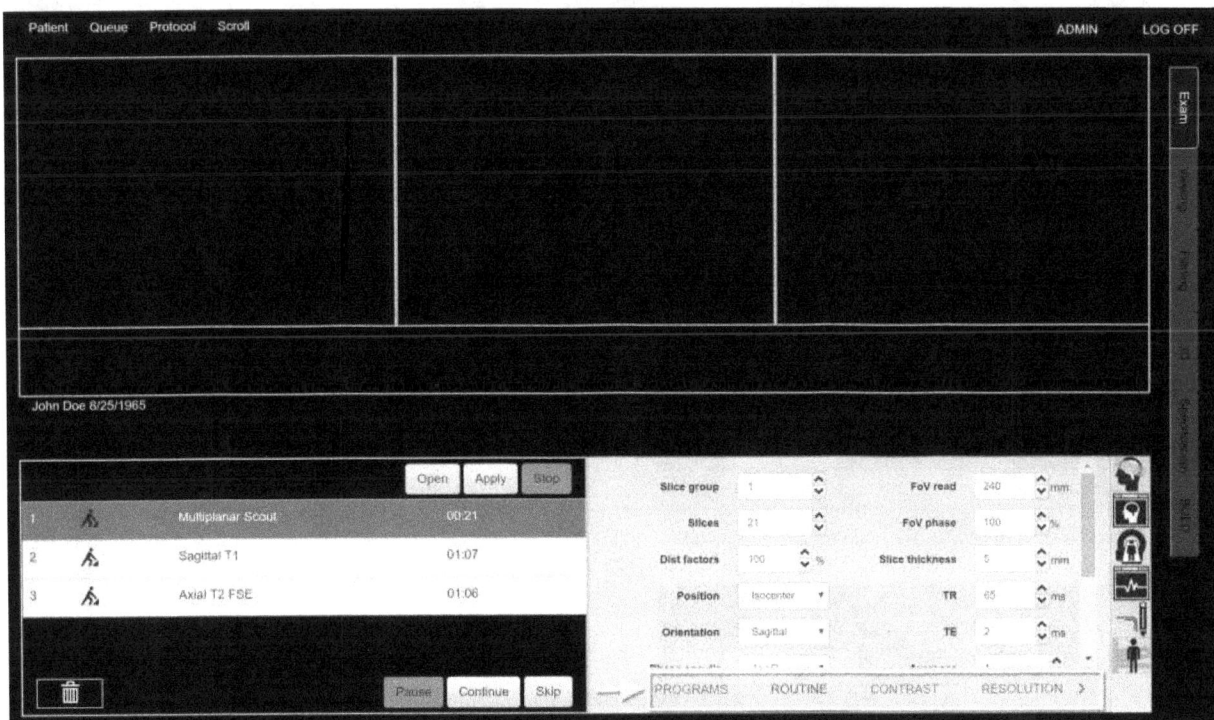

28. Apply the Parameters — Click the apply button to begin the first scan.

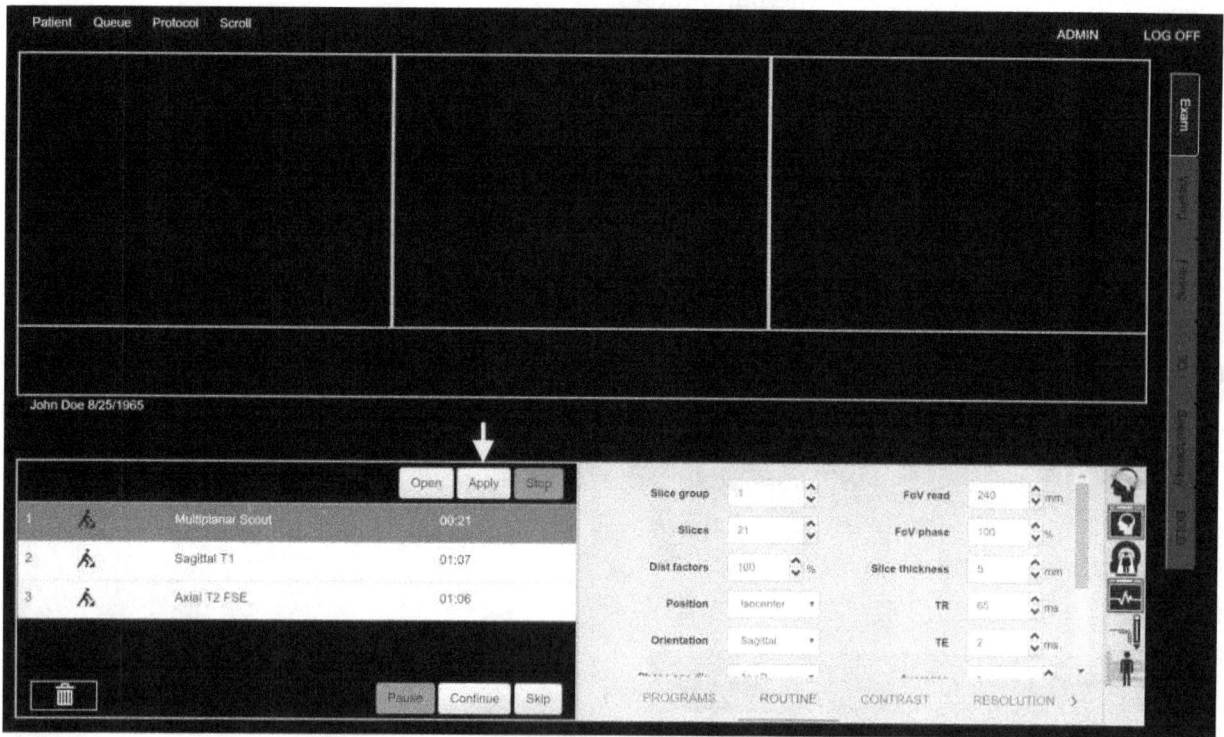

29. Image Review — Click the arrow button in the upper right corner of the view port to review the images associated with the completed scan.

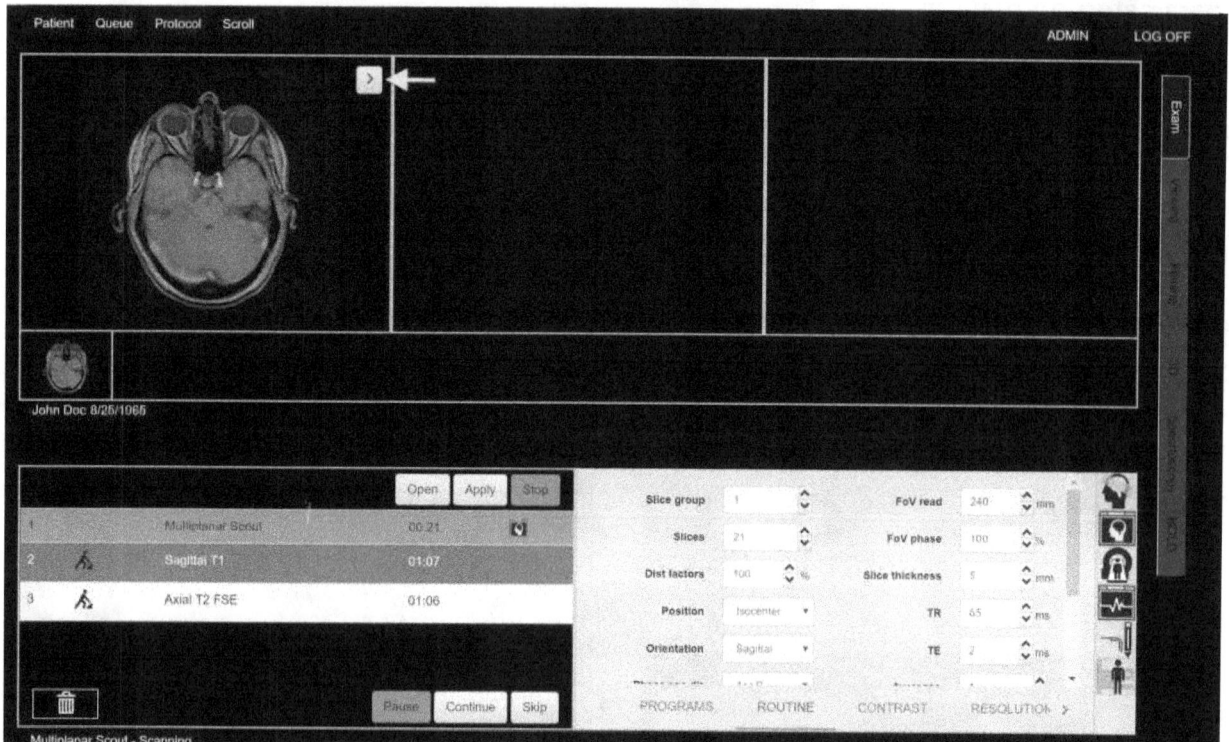

Simulator questions

1. Which area of the simulator allows you to register the patient?

_____

_____

_____

_____

_____

2. After registering the patient, which area allows you to select the protocol to be scanned?

_____

_____

_____

_____

_____

3. Once a protocol and sequence have been selected, which button allows you to view the parameter details of the sequence?

_____

_____

_____

_____

4. How can a student displayed the description of an imaging parameter and determine its

_____

_____

_____

_____

5. Once the sequence has been selected and the parameters and slices have been set up, which button allows you to scan the sequence?

_____

_____

_____

_____

_____

6. Which area of the simulator displays the images after they have been scanned?

_____

_____

_____

_____

_____

NOTES

MRI Brain Without Contrast

Objective:
In this lab you will screen the patient, scan an MRI of the brain without contrast, and evaluate the images.

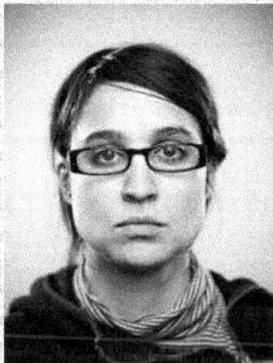

Patient Information

Patient: Johnson, Anna
Age: 25
History: 25 year old female with a history of right sided headaches times 2 weeks.
Referring Physician: Samuel Smith, MD

I. PATIENT SCREENING:
   A. Evaluate the patient requisition.
   B. Evaluate and sign the patient's screening form.
   C. Answer the patient screening questions.

II. PERFORM EXAM:
   A. If there are no contraindications, enter the patient's name and demographic information into the simulator and continue the exam performance steps. If there are contraindications, please halt the study.
   B. Select the appropriate coil.
   C. Scan the protocol listed on page 2-4. Upon the completion of each sequence evaluate the images for artifacts and pathology.
   D. Answer the procedure questions.

General Medical Center
Patient Requisition

Patient ID	Accession Number
41256832	MR1505101739

Last Name	First Name	Referring Physician
Johnson	Anna	Smith, Samuel, MD

Age	Gender	Phone	Exam
25	F	(478)555-1234	MRI Brain Without Contrast

History

25 y/o female with right sided headaches times 2 weeks.

BUN	Creatinine	GFR	
0.00	0.00	0.00	

Notes

GENERAL MEDICAL CENTER
MRI Screening Form

Patient Name: _Anna Johnson_   Sex: ☐M ☒F   Weight: _127_

Age: _25_   Referring Physician: _Dr. Samuel Smith_

Please explain the reason for which you are having an MRI exam:
Severe headaches on the right side for two weeks

Do you have or have you ever had any of the following?

☐ Yes	☒ No	Cardiac Pacemaker
☐ Yes	☒ No	Heart Surgery/Heart Valve
☐ Yes	☒ No	Implanted Cardiac Defibrillator (ICD)
☐ Yes	☒ No	Brain Surgery / Brain Aneurysm Clips
☐ Yes	☒ No	Shunts/Stents/Filters/Intravascular Coil
☐ Yes	☒ No	Eye Surgery/Implants/Spring/Wires/Retinal Tack
☐ Yes	☒ No	Eye Injury Involving Metal/Metal Shavings
☐ Yes	☒ No	Orthopedic Pins/Screws/Rods/Joints/Prosthesis
☐ Yes	☒ No	Neurostimulator / Biostimulator
☐ Yes	☒ No	Previous Neck/Back Surgery
☐ Yes	☒ No	Ear Surgery/Cochlear Implants/Hearing Aids
☐ Yes	☒ No	Vascular Access Port/Catheter
☐ Yes	☒ No	Metal Implants/Sutures/Staples or Clips
☐ Yes	☒ No	Electrical/Mechanical/Magnetic Implants
☐ Yes	☒ No	Implanted Drug Infusion Pump/Insulin Pump
☐ Yes	☒ No	Are you Pregnant?
☐ Yes	☒ No	Tattoo's/Permanent Make-up
☒ Yes	☐ No	Body Piercing, Location _Ears_
☐ Yes	☒ No	Dentures/Partials/Dental Implants
☐ Yes	☒ No	Gunshot or Shrapnel Wounds
☐ Yes	☒ No	Do you have pins in your Hair/Clothes?
☐ Yes	☒ No	Do you have Hair Extensions/Hair Pieces/Wig?
☐ Yes	☒ No	Do you have any history of kidney disease?
☐ Yes	☒ No	Do you have any history of hypertension?
☐ Yes	☒ No	Do you have any history of diabetes?

Draw the area where you are having pain.

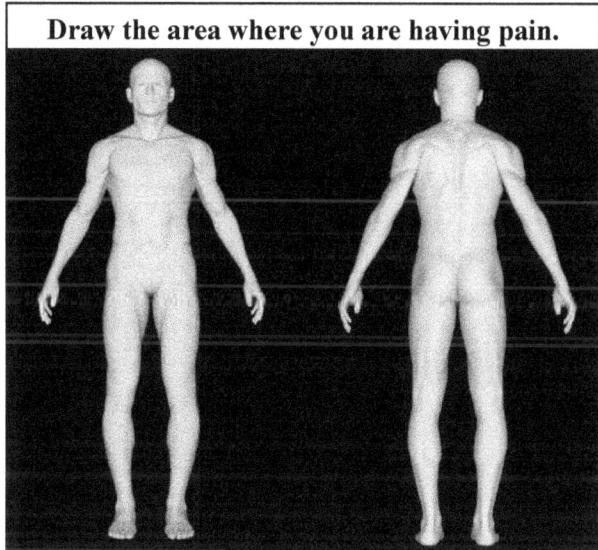

List Previous Surgeries:

None

I attest that the above information is correct to the best of my knowledge.

X _Anna Johnson_
Patient/Parent/Legal Guardian   **MRI Technologist's Signature**   **Date**

Protocol

Protocol: Brain Without Contrast

Parameters	Scout	Sagittal T1	Axial T2 FSE	Axial Flair	Axial T1	Axial DWI	Coronal T2 GRE
Patient Position	Supine	Supine	Supine	Supine	Supine	Supine	Supine
Patient Entry	Head First	Head First	Head First	Head First	Head First	Head First	Head First
Imaging Coil	Brain Coil	Brain Coil	Brain Coil	Brain Coil	Brain Coil	Brain Coil	Brain Coil
Imaging Plane	MP	Sagittal	Axial	Axial	Axial	Axial	Coronal
Pulse Sequence	T2 GRE	T1 SE	T2 FSE	FLAIR	T1 SE	DWI	T2 GRE
TR	65	550	6500	9000	400	10,000	600
TE	2	10	100	120	10	100	20
TI	0	0	0	2200	0	0	0
Flip Angle	15	90	90	90	90	90	25
ETL	0	0	16	8	0	0	0
b Value	0	0	0	0	0	1000	0
Field of View	24 cm	24 cm	24 cm	24 cm	24 cm	36 cm	24 cm
Slice Thickness	5 mm	5.0 mm	5.0 mm	5.0 mm	5.0 mm	5.0 mm	6.0 mm
Slice Spacing	5 mm	1.0 mm	1.0 mm	1.0 mm	1.0 mm	1.5 mm	1.0 mm
No. of Slices	21	20	25	25	25	25	23
Start Location	x	L 55	I 80	I 80	I 80	I 80	P 70
End Location	x	R 55	S 60	S 60	S 60	S 60	A 80
Freq. Matrix	256	256	256	256	256	128	256
Phase Matrix	128	192	256	192	256	128	192
NSA (Averages)	1	1	2	1	1	1	1
Phase Direction	1	A/P	L/R	L/R	L/R	L/R	L/R
Freq. Direction	S/I	S/I	A/P	A/P	A/P	A/P	S/I

Slice Reference

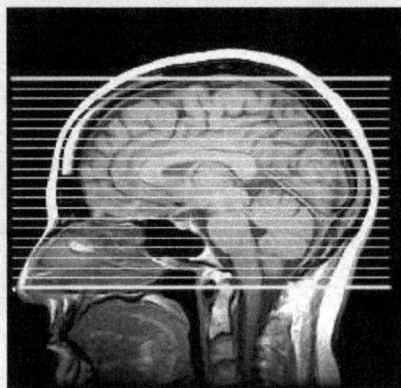

For axial images of the brain, slices should be prescribed from the foramen magnum to the vertex of the brain.

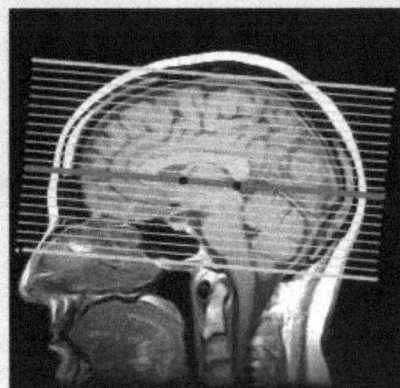

Axial slices of the brain can be planned straight or with a slight angle where the slices are parallel to anterior and posterior commissures.

Patient Screening Questions:

1. Is the exam ordered consistent with the patient's history and symptoms? If not, describe why they are not consistent.

_____

_____

_____

_____

_____

_____

_____

_____

2. Are there any contraindications that would prevent the patient from having an MRI exam? If so, list and describe each.

_____

_____

_____

_____

_____

_____

_____

_____

3. Are there any items found on the patient screening form that could cause potential artifacts? If so, please describe.

_____

_____

_____

_____

_____

_____

_____

Exam Performance Questions

4. What type of coil was selected for this procedure?

_____

_____

_____

_____

5. What is the patient's orientation?

_____

_____

_____

_____

6. Were there any artifacts on the images? If so, list the artifact name, list the sequence it appears on, describe its appearance, and define how it should be corrected.

_____

_____

_____

_____

_____

_____

_____

_____

7. Was there any pathology found on the images? If so, list the sequence it appears on and describe its appearance.

_____

_____

_____

_____

_____

_____

_____

8. If pathology was found, which of the sequences shows it best?

_____

_____

_____

_____

_____

_____

_____

_____

9. Describe why the diffusion weighted pulse sequence is commonly utilized in brain studies.

_____

_____

_____

_____

_____

_____

_____

_____

10. Using the appropriate parameters, calculate the correct scan time for the Sagittal T1 pulse sequence. See lab references VII, VIII.

_____

_____

_____

_____

_____

_____

_____

_____

NOTES

MRI Brain Without Contrast

Objective:
In this lab you will screen the patient, scan an MRI of the brain without contrast, and evaluate the images.

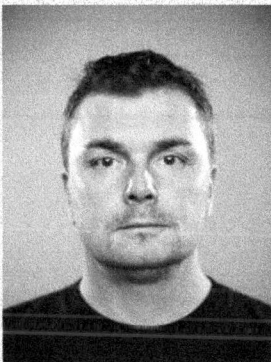

Patient Information
Patient: Davis, Jason
Age: 43
History: 43 y/o male with peripheral vision deficit and slurred speech
Referring Physician: James Wilson, MD

I. PATIENT SCREENING:
    A. Evaluate the patient requisition.
    B. Evaluate and sign the patient's screening form.
    C. Answer the patient screening questions.
    D. See reference III for lab 3.

II. PERFORM EXAM:
    A. If there are no contraindications, enter the patient's name and demographic information into the simulator and continue the exam performance steps. If there are contraindications, please halt the study.
    B. Select the appropriate coil.
    C. Scan the protocol listed on page 3 4. Upon the completion of each sequence evaluate the images for artifacts and pathology.
    D. Answer the procedure questions.

General Medical Center
Patient Requisition

Patient ID		Accession Number
5453124565		MR1505101740

Last Name	First Name	Referring Physician
Davis	Jason	Wilson, James, MD

Age	Gender	Phone		Exam
43	M	(478)555-2323		MRI Brain Without Contrast

History

43 y/o male with peripheral vision deficit and slurred speech.

BUN	Creatinine	GFR	
0.00	0.00	0.00	

Notes

GENERAL MEDICAL CENTER
MRI Screening Form

Patient Name: _TeJon Devin_   Sex: ☒M ☐F   Weight: _197_

Age: _43_   Referring Physician: _Dr. James Wilson_

Please explain the reason for which you are having an MRI exam:

Slurred speech and blurred vision

Do you have or have you ever had any of the following?

Draw the area where you are having pain.

☐ Yes ☒ No	Cardiac Pacemaker
☐ Yes ☒ No	Heart Surgery/Heart Valve
☐ Yes ☒ No	Implanted Cardiac Defibrillator (ICD)
☒ Yes ☐ No	Brain Surgery / Brain Aneurysm Clips
☐ Yes ☒ No	Shunts/Stents/Filters/Intravascular Coil
☐ Yes ☒ No	Eye Surgery/Implants/Spring/Wires/Retinal Tack
☐ Yes ☒ No	Eye Injury Involving Metal/Metal Shavings
☐ Yes ☒ No	Orthopedic Pins/Screws/Rods/Joints/Prosthesis
☐ Yes ☒ No	Neurostimulator / Biostimulator
☐ Yes ☒ No	Previous Neck/Back Surgery
☐ Yes ☒ No	Ear Surgery/Cochlear Implants/Hearing Aids
☐ Yes ☒ No	Vascular Access Port/Catheter
☐ Yes ☒ No	Metal Implants/Sutures/Staples or Clips
☐ Yes ☒ No	Electrical/Mechanical/Magnetic Implants
☐ Yes ☒ No	Implanted Drug Infusion Pump/Insulin Pump
☐ Yes ☒ No	Are you Pregnant?
☐ Yes ☒ No	Tattoo's/Permanent Make-up
☐ Yes ☒ No	Body Piercing, Location _____
☐ Yes ☒ No	Dentures/Partials/Dental Implants
☐ Yes ☒ No	Gunshot or Shrapnel Wounds
☐ Yes ☒ No	Do you have pins in your Hair/Clothes?
☐ Yes ☒ No	Do you have Hair Extensions/Hair Pieces/Wig?

☐ Yes ☒ No	Do you have any history of kidney disease?
☐ Yes ☒ No	Do you have any history of hypertension?
☐ Yes ☒ No	Do you have any history of diabetes?

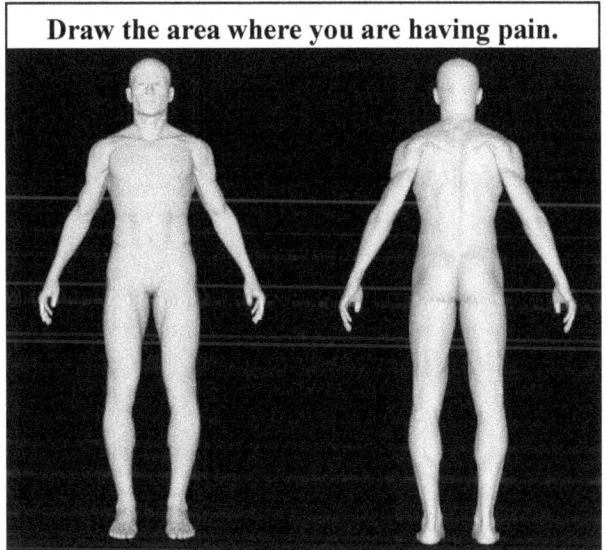

List Previous Surgeries:

Vasectomy

Gall bladder

Brain aneurysm surgery

I attest that the above information is correct to the best of my knowledge.

X _TeJon Devin_ _____   _____   _____

Patient/Parent/Legal Guardian   **MRI Technologist's Signature**   **Date**

Protocol

Protocol: Brain Without Contrast

Parameters	Scout	Sagittal T1	Axial T2 FSE	Axial Flair	Axial T1	Axial DWI	Coronal T2 GRE
Patient Position	Supine	Supine	Supine	Supine	Supine	Supine	Supine
Patient Entry	Head First	Head First	Head First	Head First	Head First	Head First	Head First
Imaging Coil	Brain Coil	Brain Coil	Brain Coil	Brain Coil	Brain Coil	Brain Coil	Brain Coil
Imaging Plane	MP	Sagittal	Axial	Axial	Axial	Axial	Coronal
Pulse Sequence	T2 GRE	T1 SE	T2 FSE	FLAIR	T1 SE	DWI	T2 GRE
TR	65	550	6500	9000	400	10,000	600
TE	2	10	100	120	10	100	20
TI	0	0	0	2200	0	0	0
Flip Angle	15	90	90	90	90	90	25
ETL	0	0	16	8	0	0	0
b Value	0	0	0	0	0	1000	0
Field of View	24 cm	24 cm	24 cm	24 cm	24 cm	36 cm	24 cm
Slice Thickness	5 mm	5.0 mm	5.0 mm	5.0 mm	5.0 mm	5.0 mm	6.0 mm
Slice Spacing	5 mm	1.0 mm	1.0 mm	1.0 mm	1.0 mm	1.5 mm	1.0 mm
No. of Slices	21	20	25	25	25	25	23
Start Location	x	L 55	I 80	I 80	I 80	I 80	P 70
End Location	x	R 55	S 60	S 60	S 60	S 60	A 80
Freq. Matrix	256	256	256	256	256	128	256
Phase Matrix	128	192	256	192	256	128	192
NSA (Averages)	1	1	2	1	1	1	1
Phase Direction	1	A/P	L/R	L/R	L/R	L/R	L/R
Freq. Direction	S/I	S/I	A/P	A/P	A/P	A/P	S/I

Slice Reference

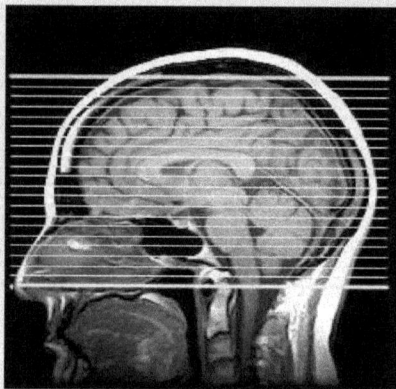

For axial images of the brain, slices should be prescribed from the foramen magnum to the vertex of the brain.

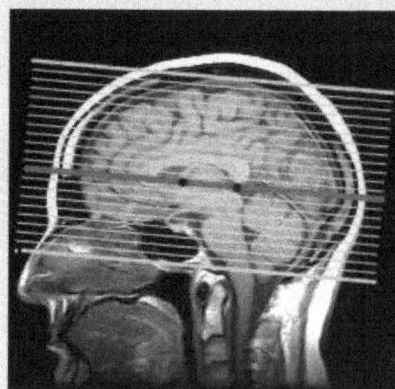

Axial slices of the brain can be planned straight or with a slight angle where the slices are parallel to anterior and posterior commissures.

Patient Screening Questions:

1. Is the exam ordered consistent with the patient's history and symptoms? If not, describe why they are not consistent.

_____
_____
_____
_____
_____
_____
_____
_____
_____

2. Are there any contraindications that would prevent the patient from having an MRI exam? If so, list and describe each.

_____
_____
_____
_____
_____
_____
_____
_____
_____

3. Are there any items found on the patient screening form that could cause potential artifacts? If so, please describe.

_____
_____
_____
_____
_____
_____
_____
_____

Exam Performance Questions

4. What type of coil was selected for this procedure?

_____

_____

_____

_____

5. What is the patient's orientation?

_____

_____

_____

_____

6. Were there any artifacts on the images? If so, list the artifact name, list the sequence it appears on, describe its appearance, and define how it should be corrected.

_____

_____

_____

_____

_____

_____

_____

_____

7. Was there any pathology found on the images? If so, list the sequence it appears on and describe its appearance.

_____

_____

_____

_____

_____

_____

_____

_____

8. Which type of image weighting is affected by changing the echo time (TE)?

_____

_____

_____

_____

_____

_____

_____

_____

9. Which imaging parameters directly affect scan time?

_____

_____

_____

_____

_____

_____

_____

_____

NOTES

MRI Brain With Contrast

Objective:

In this lab you will screen the patient, scan an MRI of the brain with contrast, and evaluate the images.

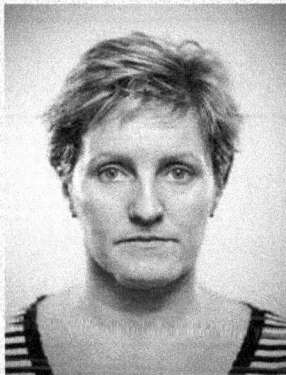

Patient Information

Patient: Hudson, Elizabeth
Age: 38
History: Evaluate for Multiple Sclerosis
Referring Physician: Winston, Harvey, MD

I. PATIENT SCREENING:

    A. Evaluate the patient requisition.
    B. Evaluate and sign the patient's screening form.
    C. Answer the patient screening questions.
    D. See lab reference I, II and VI for lab 4.

II. PERFORM EXAM:

    A. If there are no contraindications, enter the patient's name and demographic information into the simulator and continue the exam performance steps. If there are contraindications, please halt the study.
    B. Select the appropriate coil.
    C. Scan the protocol listed on page 4-4. Upon the completion of each sequence evaluate the images for artifacts and pathology.
    D. Answer the procedure questions.

General Medical Center
Patient Requisition

Patient ID			Accession Number	
3181436			MR1505101750	

Last Name		First Name	Referring Physician	
Hudson		Elizabeth	Winston, Harvey, MD	

Age	Gender	Phone	Exam
38	F	(687)555-2561	MRI Brain With Contrast

History

38 y/o female with numbness and tingling in extremities.
Evaluate for multiple sclerosis.

BUN	Creatinine	GFR	
15 mg/dL	0.75 mg/dL	105 mL/min	

Notes

GENERAL MEDICAL CENTER
MRI Screening Form

Patient Name: Elizabeth Hudson   **Sex:** ☐M ☑F   **Weight:** 145

Age: 38   **Referring Physician:** Dr. Harvey

Please explain the reason for which you are having an MRI exam:
Numbness and tingling in both arms

Do you have or have you ever had any of the following?

☐ Yes	☑No	Cardiac Pacemaker
☐ Yes	☑No	Heart Surgery/Heart Valve
☐ Yes	☑No	Implanted Cardiac Defibrillator (ICD)
☐ Yes	☑No	Brain Surgery / Brain Aneurysm Clips
☐ Yes	☑No	Shunts/Stents/Filters/Intravascular Coil
☐ Yes	☐No	Eye Surgery/Implants/Spring/Wires/Retinal Tack
☐Yes	☐No	Eye Injury Involving Metal/Metal Shavings
☐Yes	☑No	Orthopedic Pins/Screws/Rods/Joints/Prosthesis
☐Yes	☑No	Neurostimulator / Biostimulator
☐Yes	☑No	Previous Neck/Back Surgery
☐Yes	☑No	Ear Surgery/Cochlear Implants/Hearing Aids
☐Yes	☑No	Vascular Access Port/Catheter
☐Yes	☑No	Metal Implants/Sutures/Staples or Clips
☐Yes	☑No	Electrical/Mechanical/Magnetic Implants
☐Yes	☑No	Implanted Drug Infusion Pump/Insulin Pump
☐Yes	☑No	Are you Pregnant?
☐Yes	☑No	Tattoo's/Permanent Make-up
☑Yes	☐No	Body Piercing, Location Ears, Belly button
☐Yes	☑No	Dentures/Partials/Dental Implants
☐Yes	☑No	Gunshot or Shrapnel Wounds
☐Yes	☑No	Do you have pins in your Hair/Clothes?
☐Yes	☑No	Do you have Hair Extensions/Hair Pieces/Wig?
☐Yes	☑No	Do you have any history of kidney disease?
☐Yes	☑No	Do you have any history of hypertension?
☐Yes	☑No	Do you have any history of diabetes?

Draw the area where you are having pain.

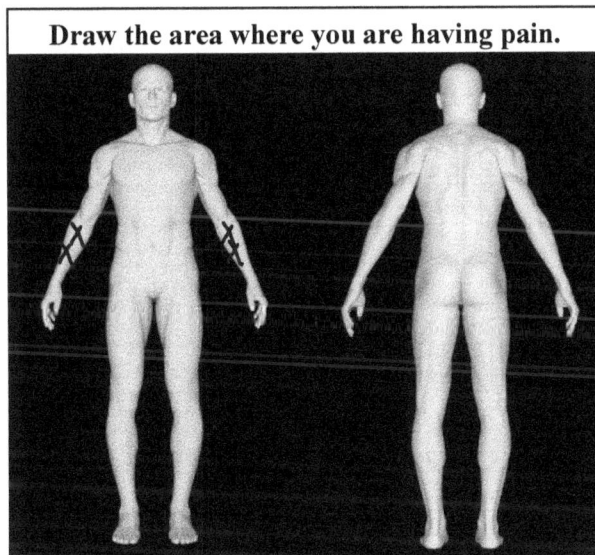

List Previous Surgeries:
None

I attest that the above information is correct to the best of my knowledge.

x Elizabeth Hudson
Patient/Parent/Legal Guardian   **MRI Technologist's Signature**   **Date**

Protocol

Protocol: Brain With Contrast

Parameters	Scout	Sagittal T1	Axial T2	Axial Flair	Axial T1	Axial DWI	Coronal T2	Sag T1 Post	Ax T1 Post
Patient Position	Supine	Supine	Supine	Supine	Supine	Supine	Supine	Supine	Supine
Patient Entry	Head First	Head First	Head First	Head First	Head First	Head First	Head First	Head First	Head First
Imaging Coil	Brain Coil	Brain Coil	Brain Coil	Brain Coil	Brain Coil	Brain Coil	Brain Coil	Brain Coil	Brain Coil
Imaging Plane	MP	Sagittal	Axial	Axial	Axial	Axial	Coronal	Sagittal	Axial
Pulse Sequence	T2 GRE	T1 SE	T2 FSE	FLAIR	T1 SE	DWI	T2 GRE	T1 SE	T1 SE
TR	65	550	6500	9000	400	10,000	600	550	400
TE	2	10	100	120	10	100	20	10	10
TI	0	0	0	2200	0	0	0	0	0
Flip Angle	15	90	90	90	90	90	25	90	90
ETL	0	0	16	8	0	0	0	0	0
b Value	0	0	0	0	0	1000	0	0	0
Field of View	24 cm	24 cm	24 cm	24 cm	24 cm	36 cm	24 cm	24 cm	24 cm
Slice Thickness	5 mm	5.0 mm	5.0 mm	5.0 mm	5.0 mm	5.0 mm	6.0 mm	5.0 mm	5.0 mm
Slice Spacing	5 mm	1.0 mm	1.0 mm	1.0 mm	1.0 mm	1.5 mm	1.0 mm	1.0 mm	1.0 mm
No. of Slices	21	20	25	25	25	25	23	20	25
Start Location	x	L 55	I 80	I 80	I 80	I 80	P 70	L 55	I 80
End Location	x	R 55	S 60	S 60	S 60	S 60	A 80	R 55	S 60
Freq. Matrix	256	256	256	256	256	128	256	256	256
Phase Matrix	128	192	256	192	256	128	192	192	256
NSA (Averages)	1	1	2	1	1	1	1	1	1
Phase Direction	X	A/P	L/R	L/R	L/R	L/R	L/R	A/P	L/R
Freq. Direction	X	S/I	A/P	A/P	A/P	A/P	S/I	S/I	A/P

Slice Reference

For axial images of the brain, slices should be prescribed from the foramen magnum to the vertex of the brain.

Axial slices of the brain can be planned straight or with a slight angle where the slices are parallel to anterior and posterior commissures.

Patient Screening Questions:

1. Is the exam ordered consistent with the patient's history and symptoms? If not, describe why they are not consistent.

_____
_____
_____
_____
_____
_____
_____
_____

2. Are there any contraindications that would prevent the patient from having an MRI exam? If so, list and describe each.

_____
_____
_____
_____
_____
_____
_____
_____

3. Are there any items found on the patient screening form that could cause potential artifacts? If so, please describe .

_____
_____
_____
_____
_____
_____
_____

Exam Performance Questions

4. What type of coil was selected for this procedure?

_____

_____

_____

_____

5. Utilizing the patient's weight and the gadolinium chart listed in the reference section, calculate the amount of contrast that should be used for the post contrast sequences. List the amount below.

_____

_____

_____

_____

6. Were there any artifacts on the images? If so, list the artifact name, list the sequence it appears on, describe its appearance, and define how it should be corrected.

_____

_____

_____

_____

_____

_____

_____

_____

7. Was there any pathology found on the images? If so, list the sequence it appears on and describe its appearance.

_____

_____

_____

_____

_____

_____

_____

_____

8. Which imaging parameter directly affects T1 weighting?

_____

_____

_____

_____

_____

_____

_____

_____

9. Which parameters directly affect image resolution?

_____

_____

_____

_____

_____

_____

_____

_____

NOTES

MRI Brain With Contrast

Objective:

In this lab you will screen the patient, scan an MRI of the brain with contrast, and evaluate the images.

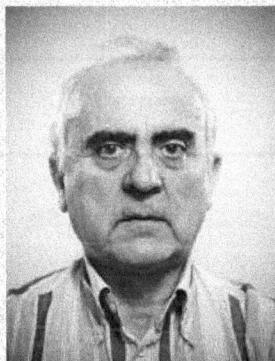

Patient Information

Patient: Cooper, Melvin
Age: 71
History: 71 y/o male with double vision and muscle weakness in the face
Referring Physician: Scott Taylor, MD

I. PATIENT SCREENING:

> A. Evaluate the patient requisition.
> B. Evaluate and sign the patient's screening form.
> C. Answer the patient screening questions.
> D. See reference I, II, and VI for the department contrast policy.
> E. See lab reference I, II and VI for lab 5.

II. PERFORM EXAM:

> A. If there are no contraindications, enter the patient's name and demographic information into the simulator and continue the exam performance steps. If there are contraindications, please halt the study.
> B. Select the appropriate coil.
> C. Scan the protocol listed on page 5-4. Upon the completion of each sequence evaluate the images for artifacts and pathology.
> D. Answer the procedure questions.

General Medical Center
Patient Requisition

Patient ID		Accession Number	
25874		MR25874195	

Last Name	First Name	Referring Physician
Cooper	Melvin	Taylor, Scott MD

Age	Gender	Phone	Exam
71	M	(478)555-7879	MRI Brain With Contrast

History

71 y/o male with double vision and muscle weakness in the face.

BUN	Creatinine	GFR	
50 mg/dL	2.4 mg/dL	12 mL/min	

Notes

GENERAL MEDICAL CENTER
MRI Screening Form

Patient Name: _Melvin Cooper_   Sex: ☒M ☐ F   Weight: _225_

Age: _71_   Referring Physician: _Dr. Scott Taylor_

Please explain the reason for which you are having an MRI exam:
Double vision and face problems

Do you have or have you ever had any of the following?

☐ Yes	☒No	Cardiac Pacemaker
☐ Yes	☒No	Heart Surgery/Heart Valve
☐ Yes	☒No	Implanted Cardiac Defibrillator (ICD)
☐ Yes	☒No	Brain Surgery / Brain Aneurysm Clips
☐ Yes	☒No	Shunts/Stents/Filters/Intravascular Coil
☐ Yes	☒No	Eye Surgery/Implants/Spring/Wires/Retinal Tack
☐Yes	☒No	Eye Injury Involving Metal/Metal Shavings
☐Yes	☒No	Orthopedic Pins/Screws/Rods/Joints/Prosthesis
☐Yes	☒No	Neurostimulator / Biostimulator
☐Yes	☒No	Previous Neck/Back Surgery
☐Yes	☒No	Ear Surgery/Cochlear Implants/Hearing Aids
☐Yes	☒No	Vascular Access Port/Catheter
☐Yes	☒No	Metal Implants/Sutures/Staples or Clips
☐Yes	☒No	Electrical/Mechanical/Magnetic Implants
☐Yes	☒No	Implanted Drug Infusion Pump/Insulin Pump
☐Yes	☒No	Are you Pregnant?
☐Yes	☒No	Tattoo's/Permanent Make-up
☐Yes	☒No	Body Piercing, Location _____
☐Yes	☒No	Dentures/Partials/Dental Implants
☐Yes	☒No	Gunshot or Shrapnel Wounds
☐Yes	☒No	Do you have pins in your Hair/Clothes?
☐Yes	☒No	Do you have Hair Extensions/Hair Pieces/Wig?
☒Yes	☐No	Do you have any history of kidney disease?
☒Yes	☐No	Do you have any history of hypertension?
☒Yes	☐No	Do you have any history of diabetes?

Draw the area where you are having pain.

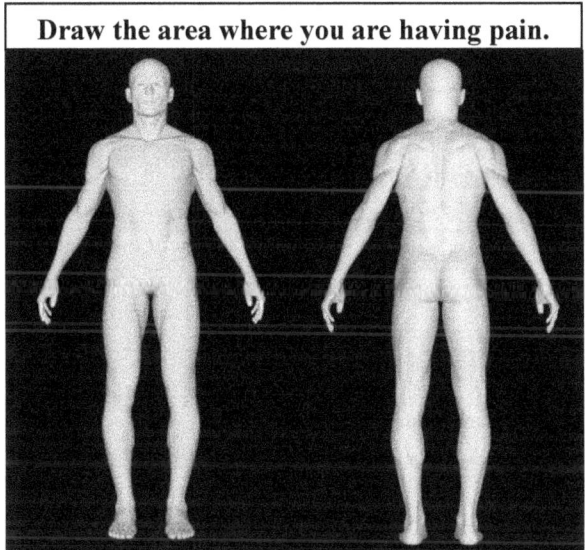

List Previous Surgeries:

None

I attest that the above information is correct to the best of my knowledge.

X_____Melvin Cooper_____   _____   _____
Patient/Parent/Legal Guardian   MRI Technologist's Signature   Date

Protocol

Protocol: Brain With Contrast

Parameters	Scout	Sagittal T1	Axial T2	Axial Flair	Axial T1	Axial DWI	Coronal T2	Sag T1 Post	Ax T1 Post
Patient Position	Supine	Supine	Supine	Supine	Supine	Supine	Supine	Supine	Supine
Patient Entry	Head First	Head First	Head First	Head First	Head First	Head First	Head First	Head First	Head First
Imaging Coil	Brain Coil	Brain Coil	Brain Coil	Brain Coil	Brain Coil	Brain Coil	Brain Coil	Brain Coil	Brain Coil
Imaging Plane	MP	Sagittal	Axial	Axial	Axial	Axial	Coronal	Sagittal	Axial
Pulse Sequence	T2 GRE	T1 SE	T2 FSE	FLAIR	T1 SE	DWI	T2 GRE	T1 SE	T1 SE
TR	65	550	6500	9000	400	10,000	600	550	400
TE	2	10	100	120	10	100	20	10	10
TI	0	0	0	2200	0	0	0	0	0
Flip Angle	15	90	90	90	90	90	25	90	90
ETL	0	0	16	8	0	0	0	0	0
b Value	0	0	0	0	0	1000	0	0	0
Field of View	24 cm	24 cm	24 cm	24 cm	24 cm	36 cm	24 cm	24 cm	24 cm
Slice Thickness	5 mm	5.0 mm	5.0 mm	5.0 mm	5.0 mm	5.0 mm	6.0 mm	5.0 mm	5.0 mm
Slice Spacing	5 mm	1.0 mm	1.0 mm	1.0 mm	1.0 mm	1.5 mm	1.0 mm	1.0 mm	1.0 mm
No. of Slices	21	20	25	25	25	25	23	20	25
Start Location	x	L 55	I 80	I 80	I 80	I 80	P 70	L 55	I 80
End Location	x	R 55	S 60	S 60	S 60	S 60	A 80	R 55	S 60
Freq. Matrix	256	256	256	256	256	128	256	256	256
Phase Matrix	128	192	256	192	256	128	192	192	256
NSA (Averages)	1	1	2	1	1	1	1	1	1
Phase Direction	X	A/P	L/R	L/R	L/R	L/R	L/R	A/P	L/R
Freq. Direction	X	S/I	A/P	A/P	A/P	A/P	S/I	S/I	A/P

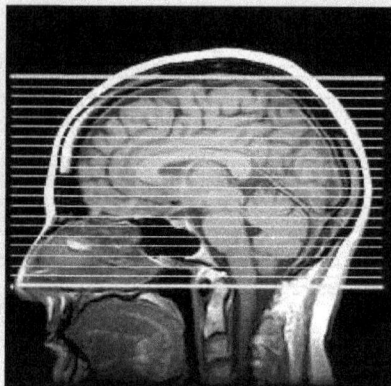

For axial images of the brain, slices should be prescribed from the foramen magnum to the vertex of the brain.

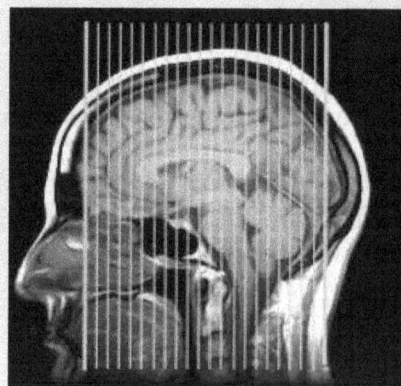

Coronal slices should be prescribed from the posterior occipital lobe to the anterior frontal lobe.

Patient Screening Questions:

1. Is the exam ordered consistent with the patient's history and symptoms? If not, describe why they are not consistent.

_____

_____

_____

_____

_____

_____

_____

_____

2. Are there any contraindications that would prevent the patient from having an MRI exam? If so, list and describe each.

_____

_____

_____

_____

_____

_____

_____

_____

_____

3. Are there any items found on the patient screening form that could cause potential artifacts? If so, please describe.

_____

_____

_____

_____

_____

_____

_____

_____

Exam Performance Questions

4. What type of coil was selected for this procedure?

_____

_____

_____

_____

_____

5. What is the patient's orientation?

_____

_____

_____

_____

_____

6. Were there any artifacts on the images? If so, list the artifact name, list the sequence it appears on, describe its appearance, and define how it should be corrected.

_____

_____

_____

_____

_____

_____

_____

_____

7. Was there any pathology found on the images? If so, list the sequence it appears on and describe its appearance.

_____

_____

_____

_____

_____

_____

_____

8. Which imaging parameters directly affect the signal-to-noise ratio?

_____

_____

_____

_____

_____

_____

_____

_____

_____

9. Describe the eGFR lab values and why they are important when screening a patient having gadolinium based contrast media.

_____

_____

_____

_____

_____

_____

_____

_____

NOTES

MRI Brain / Pituitary With Contrast

Objective:

In this lab you will screen the patient, scan an MRI of the brain and pituitary with contrast, and evaluate the images.

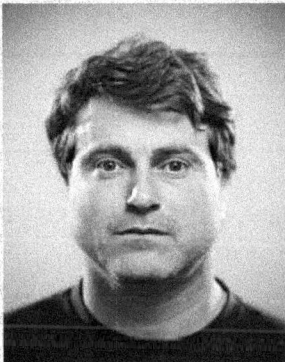

Patient Information

Patient: Frederick, Mark
Age: 32
History: 32 y/o male with Left sided Bell's palsy and excessive perspiration.
Referring Physician: Warren Walker, MD

I. PATIENT SCREENING:

    A. Evaluate the patient requisition.
    B. Evaluate and sign the patient's screening form.
    C. Answer the patient screening questions.
    D. See reference II for the department contrast policy.
    E. See lab reference I, II and VI for lab 6.

II. PERFORM EXAM:

    A. If there are no contraindications, enter the patient's name and demographic information into the simulator and continue the exam performance steps. If there are contraindications, please halt the study.
    B. Select the appropriate coil.
    C. Scan the protocol listed on page 6-4. Upon the completion of each sequence evaluate the images for artifacts and pathology.
    D. Answer the procedure questions.

General Medical Center
Patient Requisition

Patient ID		Accession Number	
41256833		MR1505101854	

Last Name	First Name	Referring Physician	
Fredrick	Mark	Walker, Warren, MD	

Age	Gender	Phone	Exam
32	M	(478)555-7706	MRI Brain/Pituitary with contrast

History

32 y/o male with Left sided Bell's palsy and excessive perspiration. R/O acromegaly.

BUN	Creatinine	GFR	
10 mg/dL	8.2 mg/dL	120 mL/min	

Notes

GENERAL MEDICAL CENTER
MRI Screening Form

Patient Name: _Mark Fredrick_   Sex: ☒ M ☐ F   Weight: _193_

Age: _32_   Referring Physician: _Dr. Warren Walker_

Please explain the reason for which you are having an MRI exam:
Face drooping and sweating a lot

Do you have or have you ever had any of the following?

☐ Yes ☒ No	Cardiac Pacemaker
☐ Yes ☒ No	Heart Surgery/Heart Valve
☐ Yes ☒ No	Implanted Cardiac Defibrillator (ICD)
☐ Yes ☒ No	Brain Surgery / Brain Aneurysm Clips
☐ Yes ☒ No	Shunts/Stents/Filters/Intravascular Coil
☒ Yes ☐ No	Eye Surgery/Implants/Spring/Wires/Retinal Tack
☐ Yes ☒ No	Eye Injury Involving Metal/Metal Shavings
☐ Yes ☒ No	Orthopedic Pins/Screws/Rods/Joints/Prosthesis
☐ Yes ☒ No	Neurostimulator / Biostimulator
☐ Yes ☒ No	Previous Neck/Back Surgery
☐ Yes ☒ No	Ear Surgery/Cochlear Implants/Hearing Aids
☐ Yes ☒ No	Vascular Access Port/Catheter
☐ Yes ☒ No	Metal Implants/Sutures/Staples or Clips
☐ Yes ☒ No	Electrical/Mechanical/Magnetic Implants
☐ Yes ☒ No	Implanted Drug Infusion Pump/Insulin Pump
☐ Yes ☒ No	Are you Pregnant?
☐ Yes ☒ No	Tattoo's/Permanent Make-up
☐ Yes ☒ No	Body Piercing, Location _____
☐ Yes ☒ No	Dentures/Partials/Dental Implants
☐ Yes ☒ No	Gunshot or Shrapnel Wounds
☐ Yes ☒ No	Do you have pins in your Hair/Clothes?
☐ Yes ☒ No	Do you have Hair Extensions/Hair Pieces/Wig?
☐ Yes ☒ No	Do you have any history of kidney disease?
☐ Yes ☒ No	Do you have any history of hypertension?
☐ Yes ☒ No	Do you have any history of diabetes?

Draw the area where you are having pain.

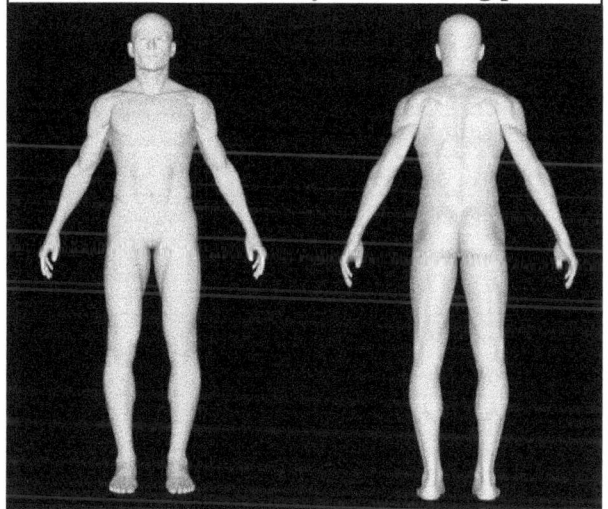

List Previous Surgeries:

Lasik eye surgery

I attest that the above information is correct to the best of my knowledge.

X _Mark Fredrick_

Patient/Parent/Legal Guardian   **MRI Technologist's Signature**   **Date**

Protocol

Protocol: Brain / Pituitary

Parameters	Scout	Coronal T2	Coronal T1 Pre Contrast	Sagittal T1 Pre Contrast	Sagittal T1 Post Contrast	Coronal T1 Post Contrast	Axial T1 Brain Post	Coronal T1 Brain Post
Patient Position	Supine	Supine	Supine	Supine	Supine	Supine	Supine	Supine
Patient Entry	Head First	Head First	Head First	Head First	Head First	Head First	Head First	Head First
Imaging Coil	Brain Coil	Brain Coil	Brain Coil	Brain Coil	Brain Coil	Brain Coil	Brain Coil	Brain Coil
Imaging Plane	MP	Coronal	Coronal	Sagittal	Sagittal	Coronal	Axial	Coronal
Pulse Sequence	T2 GRE	T2 FSE	T1 SE	T1 SE	T1 SE	T1 SE	T1 SE	T1 SE
TR	65	4000	450	450	450	450	400	650
TE	2	85	18	18	18	18	10	10
Flip Angle	15	90	90	90	90	90	90	90
ETL	0	24	0	0	0	0	0	0
Field of View	24	18 cm	18 cm	18 cm	18 cm	18 cm	22 cm	24 cm
Slice Thickness	5 mm	3.0 mm	3.0 mm	3.0 mm	3.0 mm	3.0 mm	5.0 mm	5.0 mm
Slice Spacing	5 mm	0.3 mm	0.3 mm	0.3 mm	0.3 mm	0.3 mm	1.0 mm	1.0 mm
# of Slices	21	12	12	12	12	12	25	26
Start Location	x	P19	P19	L20	L20	P19	I78	P95
End Location	x	A17	A17	R20	R20	P17	S66	A50
Freq. Matrix	256	256	256	256	256	256	256	256
Phase Matrix	128	256	192	192	192	192	192	256
NSA (Averages)	1	4	3	3	3	3	1	1
Phase Direction	1	L/R	L/R	A/P	A/P	L/R	L/R	L/R
Freq. Direction	S/I	S/I	S/I	S/I	S/I	S/I	A/P	S/I

Slice Reference

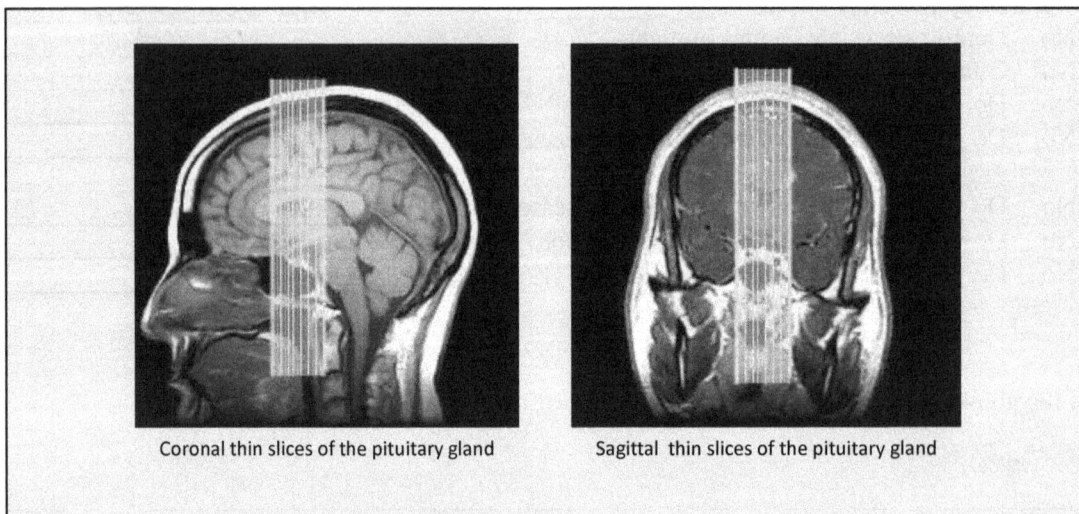

Coronal thin slices of the pituitary gland   Sagittal thin slices of the pituitary gland

Patient Screening Questions:

1. Is the exam ordered consistent with the patient's history and symptoms? If not, describe why they are not consistent.

_____

_____

_____

_____

_____

_____

_____

_____

2. Are there any contraindications that would prevent the patient from having an MRI exam? If so, list and describe each.

_____

_____

_____

_____

_____

_____

_____

_____

_____

3. Are there any items found on the patient screening form that could cause potential artifacts? If so, please describe.

_____

_____

_____

_____

_____

_____

_____

_____

Exam Performance Questions

4. What slice thickness and slice gap are used for the thin section sequences?

_____

_____

_____

_____

5. Which sequences best display the pituitary gland?

_____

_____

_____

_____

6. Were there any artifacts on the images? If so, list the artifact name, list the sequence it appears on, describe its appearance, and define how it should be corrected.

_____

_____

_____

_____

_____

_____

_____

_____

_____

7. Was there any pathology found on the images? If so, list the sequence it appears on and describe its appearance.

_____

_____

_____

_____

_____

_____

_____

_____

8. Describe why it is important to scan the pituitary gland immediately after the injection of contrast media?

_____

_____

_____

_____

_____

_____

_____

_____

9. Describe why it is common to use 1/2 dose of gadolinium based contrast media when scanning the pituitary gland.

_____

_____

_____

_____

_____

_____

_____

_____

10. Define dynamic contrast enhancement and describe how it is used during MRI imaging of the pituitary gland.

_____

_____

_____

_____

_____

_____

_____

NOTES

MRI Brain / IAC's With Contrast

Objective:

In this lab you will screen the patient, scan an MRI of the brain /IAC's with contrast, and evaluate the images.

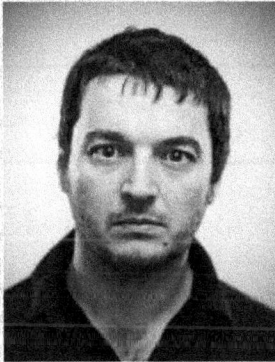

Patient Information

Patient: Adams, Alex
Age: 38
History: 38 y/o male with seizure disorder and hearing loss in the left ear.
Referring Physician: Mary Coleman, MD

I. PATIENT SCREENING:

A. Evaluate the patient requisition.
B. Evaluate and sign the patient's screening form.
C. Answer the patient screening questions.
D. See reference I, II, and VI for the department contrast policy.
E. See lab reference IV for lab 7.

II. PERFORM EXAM:

A. If there are no contraindications, enter the patient's name and demographic information into the simulator and continue the exam performance steps. If there are contraindications, please halt the study.
B. Select the appropriate coil.
C. Scan the protocol listed on page 7-4. Upon the completion of each sequence evaluate the images for artifacts and pathology.
D. Answer the procedure questions.

General Medical Center
Patient Requisition

Patient ID	Accession Number
78958	MR789582349

Last Name	First Name	Referring Physician
Adams	Alex	Coleman, Mary, MD

Age	Gender	Phone	Exam
38	M	(478)555-8808	MRI Brain and IAC's With Contrast

History

38 y/o male with seizure disorder and hearing loss in the left ear.

BUN	Creatinine	GFR	
8.0 mg/dL	1.2 mg/dL	130 mL/min	

Notes

GENERAL MEDICAL CENTER
MRI Screening Form

Patient Name: **Alex Adams**   Sex: ☒M ☐ F   Weight: **158**

Age: **38**   Referring Physician: **Dr. Mary Coleman**

Please explain the reason for which you are having an MRI exam:
Hearing loss in left ear and seizures

Do you have or have you ever had any of the following?

☐ Yes	☒No	Cardiac Pacemaker
☐ Yes	☒No	Heart Surgery/Heart Valve
☐ Yes	☒No	Implanted Cardiac Defibrillator (ICD)
☐ Yes	☒No	Brain Surgery / Brain Aneurysm Clips
☒ Yes	☐No	Shunts/Stents/Filters/Intravascular Coil
☐ Yes	☒No	Eye Surgery/Implants/Spring/Wires/Retinal Tack
☒Yes	☐No	Eye Injury Involving Metal/Metal Shavings
☐Yes	☒No	Orthopedic Pins/Screws/Rods/Joints/Prosthesis
☐Yes	☒No	Neurostimulator / Biostimulator
☐Yes	☒No	Previous Neck/Back Surgery
☐Yes	☒No	Ear Surgery/Cochlear Implants/Hearing Aids
☐Yes	☒No	Vascular Access Port/Catheter
☐Yes	☒No	Metal Implants/Sutures/Staples or Clips
☐Yes	☒No	Electrical/Mechanical/Magnetic Implants
☐Yes	☒No	Implanted Drug Infusion Pump/Insulin Pump
☐Yes	☒No	Are you Pregnant?
☐Yes	☒No	Tattoo's/Permanent Make-up
☐Yes	☒No	Body Piercing, Location _____
☐Yes	☒No	Dentures/Partials/Dental Implants
☐Yes	☒No	Gunshot or Shrapnel Wounds
☐Yes	☒No	Do you have pins in your Hair/Clothes?
☐Yes	☒No	Do you have Hair Extensions/Hair Pieces/Wig?
☐Yes	☒No	Do you have any history of kidney disease?
☐Yes	☒No	Do you have any history of hypertension?
☐Yes	☒No	Do you have any history of diabetes?

Draw the area where you are having pain.

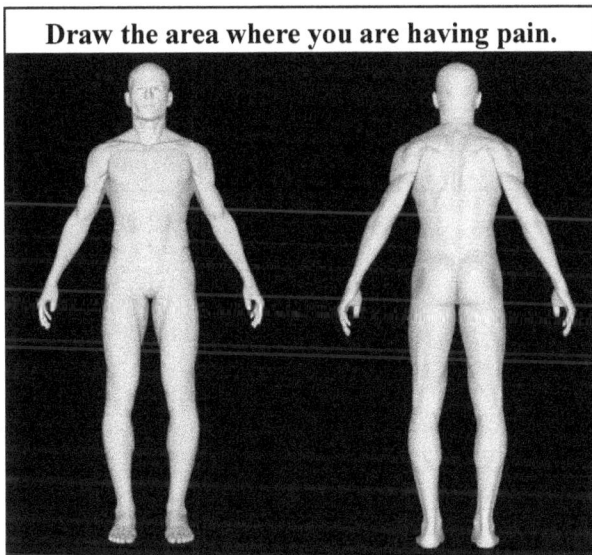

List Previous Surgeries:

Greenfield filter placement

I attest that the above information is correct to the best of my knowledge.

X **Alex Adams**
Patient/Parent/Legal Guardian   MRI Technologist's Signature   Date

Protocol

Protocol: Brain / IAC's With Contrast

Parameters	Sagittal T1	Axial T2	Axial Flair	Axial T1	Axial DWI	Coronal T2	Coronal T1 Pre	Axial T1 Pre	Axial T1 Post/FS	Axial T1 Post Brain	Coronal T1 Post/FS
Patient Position	Supine	Supine	Supine	Supine	Supine	Supine	Supine	Supine	Supine	Supine	Supine
Patient Entry	HF	HF	HF	HF	HF	HF	HF	HF	HF	HF	HF
Imaging Coil	Brain	Brain	Brain	Brain l	Brain	Brain	Brain	Brain l	Brain	Brain	Brain
Imaging Plane	Sagittal	Axial	Axial	Axial	Axial	Coronal	Coronal	Axial	Axial	Axial	Coronal
Pulse Sequence	T1 SE	T2 FSE	FLAIR	T1 SE	DWI	T2 FSE	T1 SE	T1 SE	T1 FSE	T1 SE	T1 SE
TR	550	6500	9000	400	10,000	4900	450	450	420	400	450
TE	10	100	120	10	100	85	14	14	8	10	14
TI	0	0	2200	0	0	0	0	0	0	0	0
Flip Angle	90	90	90	90	90	90	90	90	90	90	90
ETL	0	16	8	0	0	16	0	0	3	0	0
b Value	0	0	0	0	1000	0	0	0	0	0	0
Field of View	24 cm	24 cm	24 cm	24 cm	36 cm	18 cm	18 cm	18 cm	18 cm	22 cm	18 cm
Slice Thickness	5.0 mm	5.0 mm	5.0 mm	5.0 mm	5.0 mm	3.0 mm	3.0 mm	3.0 mm	3.0 mm	5.0 mm	3.0 mm
Slice Spacing	1.0 mm	1.0 mm	1.0 mm	1.0 mm	1.5 mm	0.5 mm	0.0 mm	0.0 mm	0.0 mm	1.0 mm	0.0 mm
No. of Slices	20	25	25	25	25	12	12	12	12	25	12
Start Location	L 55	I 80	I 80	I 80	I 80	P47	P44	I32	I32	I45	P44
End Location	R 55	S 60	S 60	S 60	S 60	P9	P11	S1	S1	S98	P11
Freq. Matrix	256	256	256	256	128	256	256	256	256	256	256
Phase Matrix	192	256	192	256	128	256	224	224	224	256	224
NSA (Averages)	1	2	1	1	1	2	2	2	2	2	2
Phase Direction	A/P	L/R	L/R	L/R	L/R	L/R	L/R	L/R	L/R	L/R	L/R
Freq. Direction	S/I	A/P	A/P	A/P	A/P	S/I	S/I	A/P	A/P	A/P	S/I

Slice Reference

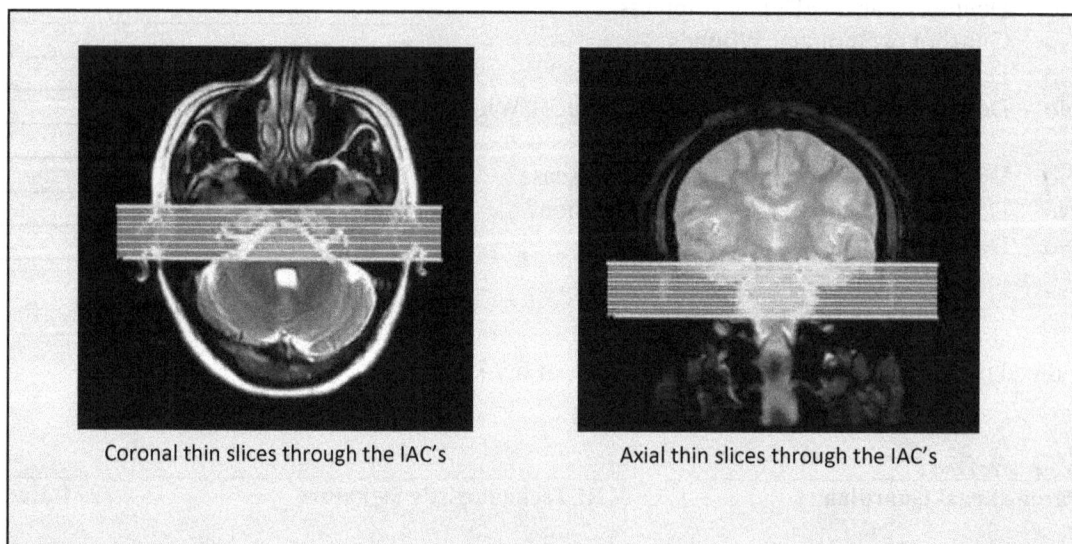

Coronal thin slices through the IAC's

Axial thin slices through the IAC's

Patient Screening Questions:

1. Is the exam ordered consistent with the patient's history and symptoms? If not, describe why they are not consistent.

_____

_____

_____

_____

_____

_____

_____

_____

2. Are there any contraindications that would prevent the patient from having an MRI exam? If so, list and describe each.

_____

_____

_____

_____

_____

_____

_____

_____

3. Are there any items found on the patient screening form that could cause potential artifacts? If so, please describe.

_____

_____

_____

_____

_____

_____

_____

Exam Performance Questions

4. MRI procedures of the internal auditory canal image which cranial nerve?

_____

_____

_____

_____

5. Which sequences best display the nerves of the internal auditory canal?

_____

_____

_____

_____

6. Were there any artifacts on the images? If so, list the artifact name, list the sequence it appears on, describe its appearance, and define how it should be corrected.

_____

_____

_____

_____

_____

_____

_____

_____

_____

7. Was there any pathology found on the images? If so, list the sequence it appears on and describe its appearance.

_____

_____

_____

_____

_____

_____

_____

_____

8. Describe when it would be beneficial to angle the thin slice sequences when imaging the internal auditory canal?.

_____

_____

_____

_____

_____

_____

_____

_____

_____

9. Describe how slice thickness affects the signal to noise ratio.

_____

_____

_____

_____

_____

_____

_____

_____

NOTES

MRI Brain / Orbit With Contrast

Objective:

In this lab you will screen the patient, scan an MRI of the brain /orbits with contrast, and evaluate the images.

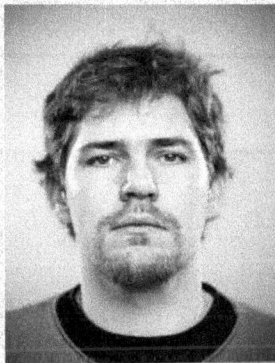

Patient Information

Patient: Anderson, William
Age: 24
History: 24 y/o male with palpable edema in the left orbit.
Referring Physician: Robert Cantrell, MD

I. PATIENT SCREENING:

A. Evaluate the patient requisition.
B. Evaluate and sign the patient's screening form.
C. Answer the patient screening questions.
D. See reference I, II, and VI for the department contrast policy.

II. PERFORM EXAM:

A. If there are no contraindications, enter the patient's name and demographic information into the simulator and continue the exam performance steps. If there are contraindications, please halt the study.
B. Select the appropriate coil.
C. Scan the protocol listed on page 8-4. Upon the completion of each sequence evaluate the images for artifacts and pathology.
D. Answer the procedure questions.

General Medical Center
Patient Requisition

Patient ID			Accession Number	
45968			MR459685462	

Last Name		First Name	Referring Physician	
Anderson		William	Cantrell, Robert, MD	

Age	Gender	Phone	Exam
24	M	(478)555-8808	MRI Brain / Orbits With Contrast

History

24 y/o male with palpable edema in the right orbit.

BUN	Creatinine	GFR	
12.0 mg/dL	.90 mg/dL	99 mL/min	

Notes

GENERAL MEDICAL CENTER
MRI Screening Form

Patient Name: _William Anderson_   Sex: ☒M ☐ F Weight: _205_

Age: _24_   Referring Physician: _Dr. Robert Cantrell_

Please explain the reason for which you are having an MRI exam:

Pain and swelling in left eye.

Do you have or have you ever had any of the following?

☐ Yes	☒No	Cardiac Pacemaker
☐ Yes	☒No	Heart Surgery/Heart Valve
☐ Yes	☒No	Implanted Cardiac Defibrillator (ICD)
☐ Yes	☒No	Brain Surgery / Brain Aneurysm Clips
☐ Yes	☒No	Shunts/Stents/Filters/Intravascular Coil
☐ Yes	☒No	Eye Surgery/Implants/Spring/Wires/Retinal Tack
☐ Yes	☒No	Eye Injury Involving Metal/Metal Shavings
☐ Yes	☒No	Orthopedic Pins/Screws/Rods/Joints/Prosthesis
☐ Yes	☒No	Neurostimulator / Biostimulator
☐ Yes	☒No	Previous Neck/Back Surgery
☐ Yes	☒No	Ear Surgery/Cochlear Implants/Hearing Aids
☐ Yes	☒No	Vascular Access Port/Catheter
☐ Yes	☒No	Metal Implants/Sutures/Staples or Clips
☐ Yes	☒No	Electrical/Mechanical/Magnetic Implants
☐ Yes	☒No	Implanted Drug Infusion Pump/Insulin Pump
☐ Yes	☒No	Are you Pregnant?
☐ Yes	☒No	Tattoo's/Permanent Make-up
☐ Yes	☒No	Body Piercing, Location _____
☐ Yes	☒No	Dentures/Partials/Dental Implants
☐ Yes	☒No	Gunshot or Shrapnel Wounds
☐ Yes	☒No	Do you have pins in your Hair/Clothes?
☐ Yes	☒No	Do you have Hair Extensions/Hair Pieces/Wig?
☐ Yes	☒No	Do you have any history of kidney disease?
☐ Yes	☒No	Do you have any history of hypertension?
☐ Yes	☒No	Do you have any history of diabetes?

Draw the area where you are having pain.

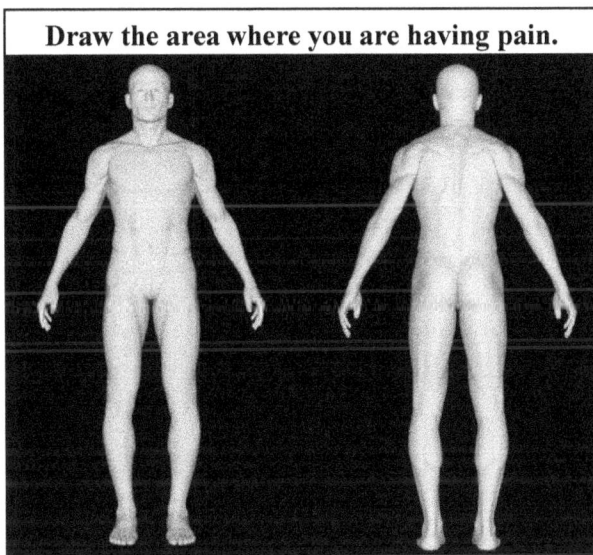

List Previous Surgeries:

None

I attest that the above information is correct to the best of my knowledge.

X___William Anderson_____   _____   _____
Patient/Parent/Legal Guardian   **MRI Technologist's Signature**   **Date**

Protocol

Protocol: Brain/ Orbit With Contrast

Parameters	Scout	Sagittal T2	Axial T1 Pre	Coronal T1 Pre	Coronal T1 Post	Axial T1 Post
Patient Position	Supine	Supine	Supine	Supine	Supine	Supine
Patient Entry	Head First	Head First	Head First	Head First	Head First	Head First
Imaging Coil	Brain Coil	Brain Coil	Brain Coil	Brain Coil	Brain Coil	Brain Coil
Imaging Plane	MP	Sagittal	Axial	Coronal	Coronal	Axial
Pulse Sequence	T2 GRE	T2 FSE	T1 SE	T1 SE	T1 SE	T1 SE
TR	65	4000	450	350	350	450
TE	2	103	14	14	14	14
TI	0	0	0	0	0	0
Flip Angle	15	90	90	90	90	90
ETL	0	16	0	0	0	0
Field of View	24 cm	24 cm	16 cm	16 cm	16 cm	16 cm
Slice Thickness	5 mm	5.0 mm	3.0 mm	4.0 mm	4.0 mm	3.0 mm
Slice Spacing	5 mm	1.0 mm	0.0 mm	0.5 mm	0.5 mm	0.0 mm
Number of Slices	21	20	14	22	22	14
Start Location	x	L 55	I40	P35	P35	I40
End Location	x	R 55	I2	A60	A60	I2
Freq. Matrix	256	256	256	256	256	256
Phase Matrix	128	192	224	224	224	224
NSA (Averages)	1	1	2	2	2	2
Phase Direction	1	A/P	L/R	L/R	L/R	L/R
Freq. Direction	S/I	S/I	A/P	A/P	A/P	A/P

Slice Reference

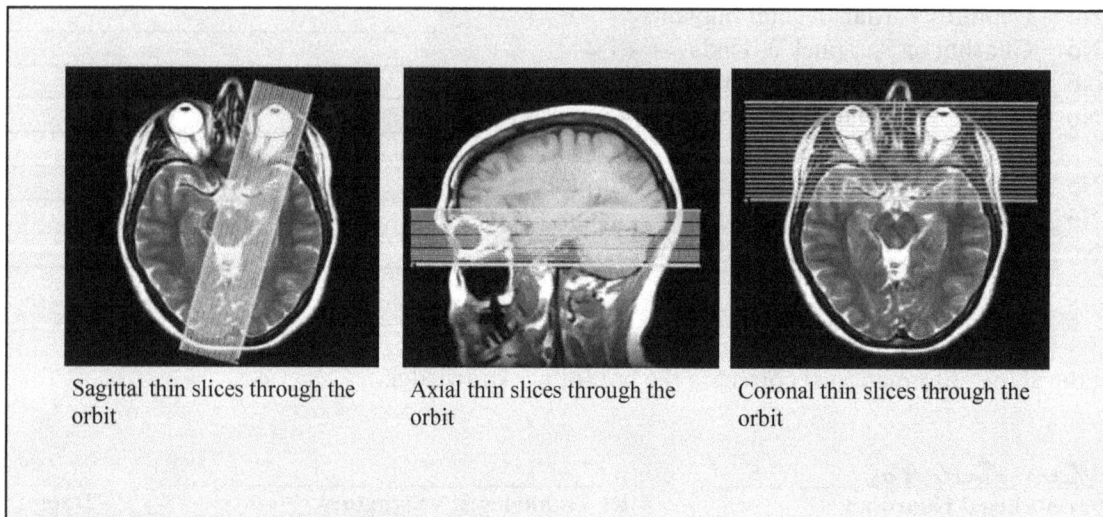

Sagittal thin slices through the orbit

Axial thin slices through the orbit

Coronal thin slices through the orbit

Patient Screening Questions:

1. Is the exam ordered consistent with the patient's history and symptoms? If not, describe why they are not consistent.

_____

_____

_____

_____

_____

_____

_____

_____

2. Are there any contraindications that would prevent the patient from having an MRI exam? If so, list and describe each.

_____

_____

_____

_____

_____

_____

_____

_____

_____

3. Are there any items found on the patient screening form that could cause potential artifacts? If so, please describe.

_____

_____

_____

_____

_____

_____

_____

_____

Exam Performance Questions

4. Which cranial nerve is the optic nerve?

_____

_____

_____

_____

5. Which sequence(s) best display the optic nerves?

_____

_____

_____

_____

6. Were there any artifacts on the images? If so, list the artifact name, list the sequence it appears on, describe its appearance, and define how it should be corrected.

_____

_____

_____

_____

_____

_____

_____

_____

7. Was there any pathology found on the images? If so, list the sequence it appears on and describe its appearance.

_____

_____

_____

_____

_____

_____

_____

8. Describe why it is important for the patient to close their eyes during an MRI of the orbits.

_____

_____

_____

_____

_____

_____

_____

_____

9. Describe why it is important to have female patients remove makeup (specifically mascara) before an examination of the orbits.

_____

_____

_____

_____

_____

_____

_____

_____

10. Describe why the saturation of fat is important to diagnosing pathology during an MRI examination of the orbits.

_____

_____

_____

_____

_____

_____

_____

_____

NOTES

MRI Cervical Spine

Objective:

In this lab you will screen the patient, scan an MRI of the cervical spine without contrast, and evaluate the images.

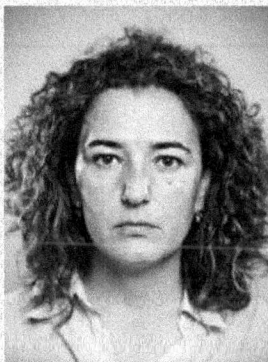

Patient Information

Patient: Swanson, Mary
Age: 45
History: 45 y/o female with history of neck pain with left sided radiculopathy
Referring Physician: Frank Everett, MD

I. PATIENT SCREENING:

A. Evaluate the patient requisition.
B. Evaluate and sign the patient's screening form.
C. Answer the patient screening questions.

II. PERFORM EXAM:

A. If there are no contraindications, enter the patient's name and demographic information into the simulator and continue the exam performance steps. If there are contraindications, please halt the study.
B. Select the appropriate coil.
C. Scan the protocol listed on page 9-4. Upon the completion of each sequence evaluate the images for artifacts and pathology.
D. Answer the procedure questions.

General Medical Center Patient Requisition				
Patient ID 55216			**Accession Number** MR5521633	
Last Name Swanson		**First Name** Mary	**Referring Physician** Everett, Frank, MD	
Age 45	**Gender** F	**Phone** (478)555-9909	**Exam** MRI C-Spine Without Contrast	
History 45 y/o female with history of neck pain with left sided radiculopathy.				
BUN 0.00	**Creatinine** 0.00	**GFR** 0.00		
Notes				

GENERAL MEDICAL CENTER
MRI Screening Form

Patient Name: _Mary Swanson_   Sex: ☐M ☒F   Weight: 125

Age: 45   Referring Physician: _Dr. Frank Everett_

Please explain the reason for which you are having an MRI exam:
Neck pain and numbness on the left side

Do you have or have you ever had any of the following?

☐ Yes	☒No	Cardiac Pacemaker
☐ Yes	☒No	Heart Surgery/Heart Valve
☐ Yes	☒No	Implanted Cardiac Defibrillator (ICD)
☐ Yes	☒No	Brain Surgery / Brain Aneurysm Clips
☐ Yes	☒No	Shunts/Stents/Filters/Intravascular Coil
☐ Yes	☒No	Eye Surgery/Implants/Spring/Wires/Retinal Tack
☐ Yes	☒No	Eye Injury Involving Metal/Metal Shavings
☐ Yes	☒No	Orthopedic Pins/Screws/Rods/Joints/Prosthesis
☐ Yes	☒No	Neurostimulator / Biostimulator
☐ Yes	☒No	Previous Neck/Back Surgery
☐ Yes	☒No	Ear Surgery/Cochlear Implants/Hearing Aids
☐ Yes	☒No	Vascular Access Port/Catheter
☐ Yes	☒No	Metal Implants/Sutures/Staples or Clips
☐ Yes	☒No	Electrical/Mechanical/Magnetic Implants
☐ Yes	☒No	Implanted Drug Infusion Pump/Insulin Pump
☐ Yes	☒No	Are you Pregnant?
☐ Yes	☒No	Tattoo's/Permanent Make-up
☒Yes	☐No	Body Piercing, Location _Ears, Belly button_
☐ Yes	☒No	Dentures/Partials/Dental Implants
☐ Yes	☒No	Gunshot or Shrapnel Wounds
☐ Yes	☒No	Do you have pins in your Hair/Clothes?
☐ Yes	☒No	Do you have Hair Extensions/Hair Pieces/Wig?
☐ Yes	☒No	Do you have any history of kidney disease?
☐ Yes	☒No	Do you have any history of hypertension?
☐ Yes	☒No	Do you have any history of diabetes?

Draw the area where you are having pain.

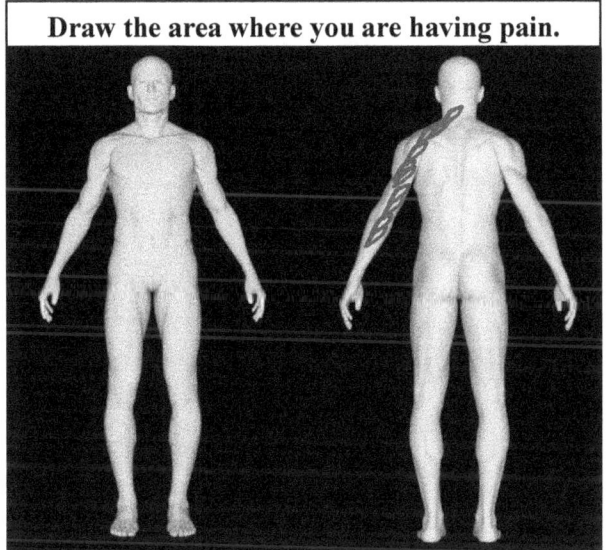

List Previous Surgeries:

Hysterectomy

Appendectomy

I attest that the above information is correct to the best of my knowledge.

X _Mary Swanson_
Patient/Parent/Legal Guardian   **MRI Technologist's Signature**   **Date**

Protocol

C-Spine without contrast

Parameters	Sagittal T1	Sagittal T2	Axial T2
Patient Position	Supine	Supine	Supine
Patient Entry	Head First	Head First	Head First
Imaging Coil	CTL Spine Coil	CTL Spine Coil	CTL Spine Coil
Imaging Plane	Sagittal	Sagittal	Axial
Pulse Sequence	T1 SE	T2 FSE	T2 GRE
TR	450	3300	700
TE	15	110	17
Flip Angle	90	90	30
Echo Train Length	0	32	0
Field of View	24 cm	24 cm	20 cm
Slice Thickness	3.0 mm	3.0 mm	4.0 mm
Slice Spacing	1.0 mm	1.0 mm	1.0 mm
Number of Slices	11	11	21
Start Location	L-20	L-20	S-26
End Location	R-20	R-20	I-73
Freq. Matrix	256	512	256
Phase Matrix	256	512	192
NSA (Averages)	2	2	2
Phase Direction	A/P	A/P	A/P
Freq. Direction	S/I	S/I	L/R

Slice Reference

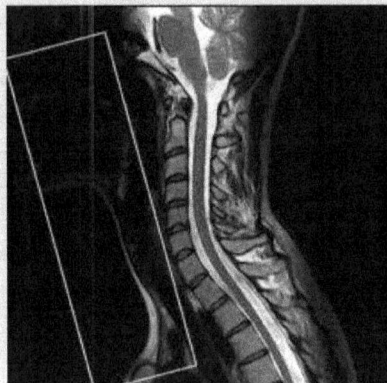

Presaturation pulses can be utilized to minimize motion caused by swallowing.

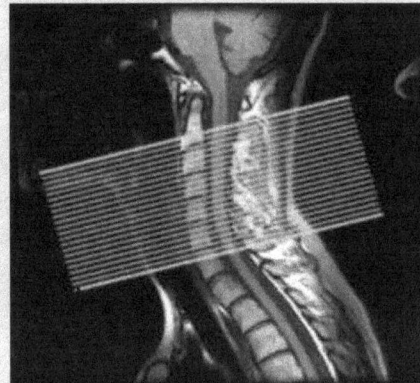

Axial slices should be prescribed so that there is a general angle through the disk spaces.

Patient Screening Questions:

1. Is the exam ordered consistent with the patient's history and symptoms? If not, describe why they are not consistent.

_____

_____

_____

_____

_____

_____

_____

_____

2. Are there any contraindications that would prevent the patient from having an MRI exam? If so, list and describe each.

_____

_____

_____

_____

_____

_____

_____

_____

3. Are there any items found on the patient screening form that could cause potential artifacts? If so, please describe.

_____

_____

_____

_____

_____

_____

_____

Exam Performance Questions

4. What type of coil was selected for this procedure?

_____

_____

_____

_____

5. What is the patient's orientation?

_____

_____

_____

_____

6. Were there any artifacts on the images? If so, list the artifact name, list the sequence it appears on, describe its appearance, and define how it should be corrected.

_____

_____

_____

_____

_____

_____

_____

_____

7. Was there any pathology found on the images? If so, list the sequence it appears on and describe its appearance.

_____

_____

_____

_____

_____

_____

_____

_____

8. Describe why it is important to begin with the number two when counting the vertebral bodies on a sagittal image of the cervical spine.

_____

_____

_____

_____

_____

_____

_____

_____

9. Describe why an anterior saturation pulse is often utilized on procedures of the cervical spine.

_____

_____

_____

_____

_____

_____

_____

_____

10. Describe how the field-of-view affects both the signal to noise ratio and spatial resolution.

_____

_____

_____

_____

_____

_____

_____

_____

NOTES

MRI Cervical Spine With Contrast

Objective:

In this lab you will screen the patient, scan an MRI of the cervical spine with contrast, and evaluate the images.

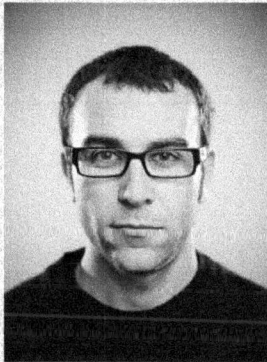

Patient Information

Patient: Moore, Fred
Age: 37
History: 37 y/o male with brachial neuritis and transverse myelitis.
Referring Physician: Wade Howard, MD

I. PATIENT SCREENING:

A. Evaluate the patient requisition.
B. Evaluate and sign the patient's screening form.
C. Answer the patient screening questions.
D. See reference I, II, and VI for the department contrast policy.

II. PERFORM EXAM:

A. If there are no contraindications, enter the patient's name and demographic information into the simulator and continue the exam performance steps. If there are contraindications, please halt the study.
B. Select the appropriate coil.
C. Scan the protocol listed on page 10-4. Upon the completion of each sequence evaluate the images for artifacts and pathology.
D. Answer the procedure questions.

General Medical Center
Patient Requisition

Patient ID			Accession Number	
65897			MR658977453	

Last Name		First Name	Referring Physician	
Moore		Fred	Howard, Wade, MD	

Age	Gender	Phone		Exam
37	M	(478)555-1010		MRI C-Spine With Contrast

History

37 y/o male with brachial neuritis and transverse myelitis.

BUN	Creatinine	GFR	
14 mg/mL	1.2 mg/mL	120 mL/min	

Notes

GENERAL MEDICAL CENTER
MRI Screening Form

Patient Name: _Fred Moore_   **Sex:** ☐M ☒F   **Weight:** _189_

Age: _37_   **Referring Physician:** _Dr. Wade Howard_

Please explain the reason for which you are having an MRI exam:
Tingling and burning in the neck shoulders and arms

Do you have or have you ever had any of the following?

☐ Yes	☒ No	Cardiac Pacemaker
☐ Yes	☒ No	Heart Surgery/Heart Valve
☐ Yes	☒ No	Implanted Cardiac Defibrillator (ICD)
☐ Yes	☒ No	Brain Surgery / Brain Aneurysm Clips
☐ Yes	☒ No	Shunts/Stents/Filters/Intravascular Coil
☐ Yes	☒ No	Eye Surgery/Implants/Spring/Wires/Retinal Tack
☐ Yes	☒ No	Eye Injury Involving Metal/Metal Shavings
☐ Yes	☒ No	Orthopedic Pins/Screws/Rods/Joints/Prosthesis
☐ Yes	☒ No	Neurostimulator / Biostimulator
☐ Yes	☒ No	Previous Neck/Back Surgery
☐ Yes	☒ No	Ear Surgery/Cochlear Implants/Hearing Aids
☐ Yes	☒ No	Vascular Access Port/Catheter
☐ Yes	☒ No	Metal Implants/Sutures/Staples or Clips
☐ Yes	☒ No	Electrical/Mechanical/Magnetic Implants
☐ Yes	☒ No	Implanted Drug Infusion Pump/Insulin Pump
☐ Yes	☒ No	Are you Pregnant?
☐ Yes	☒ No	Tattoo's/Permanent Make-up
☐ Yes	☒ No	Body Piercing, Location _____
☐ Yes	☒ No	Dentures/Partials/Dental Implants
☐ Yes	☒ No	Gunshot or Shrapnel Wounds
☐ Yes	☒ No	Do you have pins in your Hair/Clothes?
☐ Yes	☒ No	Do you have Hair Extensions/Hair Pieces/Wig?
☐ Yes	☒ No	Do you have any history of kidney disease?
☐ Yes	☒ No	Do you have any history of hypertension?
☒ Yes	☐ No	Do you have any history of diabetes?

Draw the area where you are having pain.

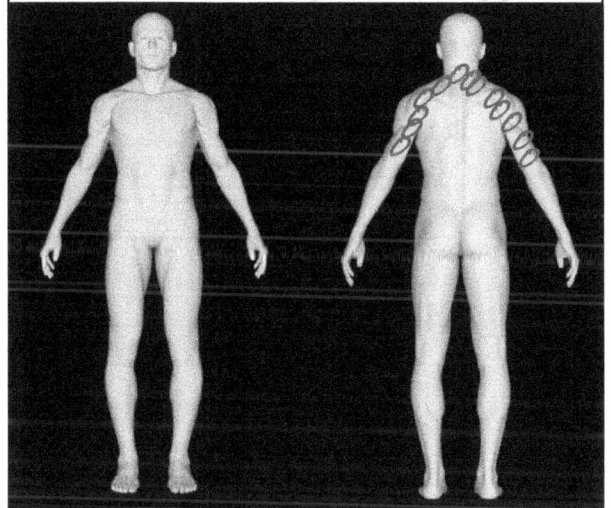

List Previous Surgeries:

None

I attest that the above information is correct to the best of my knowledge.

X _Fred Moore_ _____   _____   _____
Patient/Parent/Legal Guardian   **MRI Technologist's Signature**   **Date**

Protocol

Protocol: C-Spine With Contrast

Parameters	Sagittal T1	Sagittal T2	Axial T2	Sagittal T1 Post	Axial T1 Post
Patient Position	Supine	Supine	Supine	Supine	Supine
Patient Entry	Head First	Head First	Head First	Head First	Head First
Imaging Coil	CTL Spine Coil	CTL Spine Coil	CTL Spine Coil	CTL Spine Coil	CTL Spine Coil
Imaging Plane	Sagittal	Sagittal	Axial	Sagittal	Axial
Pulse Sequence	T1 SE	T2 FSE	T2 GRE	T1 SE	T1 SE
TR	450	3300	700	450	450
TE	15	110	17	15	15
Flip Angle	90	90	30	90	90
ETL	0	32	0	0	0
Field of View	24 cm	24 cm	20 cm	24 cm	20 cm
Slice Thickness	3.0 mm	3.0 mm	4.0 mm	3.0 mm	4.0 mm
Slice Spacing	1.0 mm	1.0 mm	1.0 mm	1.0 mm	1.0 mm
No. of Slices	11	11	21	11	21
Start Location	L-20	L-20	S-26	L-20	S-26
End Location	R-20	R-20	I-73	R-20	I-73
Freq. Matrix	256	512	256	256	256
Phase Matrix	256	512	192	256	256
NSA (Averages)	2	2	2	2	2
Phase Direction	A/P	A/P	A/P	A/P	A/P
Freq. Direction	S/I	S/I	L/R	S/I	L/R

Slice Reference

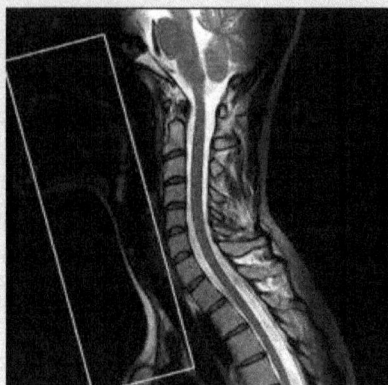

Presaturation pulses can be utilized to minimize motion caused by swallowing.

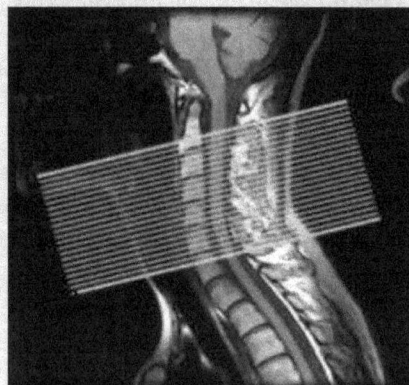

Axial slices should be prescribed so that there is a general angle through the disk spaces.

Patient Screening Questions:

1. Is the exam ordered consistent with the patient's history and symptoms? If not, describe why they are not consistent.

_____
_____
_____
_____
_____
_____
_____
_____
_____

2. Are there any contraindications that would prevent the patient from having an MRI exam? If so, list and describe each.

_____
_____
_____
_____
_____
_____
_____
_____
_____

3. Are there any items found on the patient screening form that could cause potential artifacts? If so, please describe .

_____
_____
_____
_____
_____
_____
_____
_____

Exam Performance Questions

4. What type of coil was selected for this procedure?

_____

_____

_____

_____

5. What is the patient's orientation?

_____

_____

_____

_____

6. Were there any artifacts on the images? If so, list the artifact name, list the sequence it appears on, describe its appearance, and define how it should be corrected.

_____

_____

_____

_____

_____

_____

_____

_____

7. Was there any pathology found on the images? If so, list the sequence it appears on and describe its appearance.

_____

_____

_____

_____

_____

_____

_____

_____

8. Describe how TR or repetition time affects the signal to noise ratio.

_____

_____

_____

_____

_____

_____

_____

_____

NOTES

MRI Lumbar Spine

Objective:

In this lab you will screen the patient, scan an MRI of the Lumbar spine without contrast, and evaluate the images.

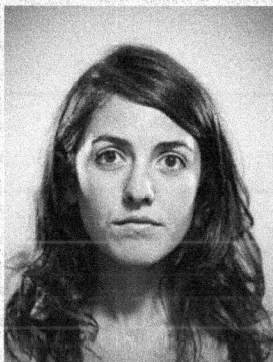

> ## Patient Information
>
> **Patient:** Smith, Andrea
> **Age:** 34
> **History:** 34 y/o female with LBP and numbness in the left lower extremity.
> **Referring Physician:** Wilson Fox, MD

I. PATIENT SCREENING:

A. Evaluate the patient requisition.
B. Evaluate and sign the patient's screening form.
C. Answer the patient screening questions.

II. PERFORM EXAM:

A. If there are no contraindications, enter the patient's name and demographic information into the simulator and continue the exam performance steps. If there are contraindications, please halt the study.
B. Select the appropriate coil.
C. Scan the protocol listed on page 11-4. Upon the completion of each sequence evaluate the images for artifacts and pathology.
D. Answer the procedure questions.

General Medical Center
Patient Requisition

Patient ID			Accession Number	
33598			MR33598803	

Last Name		First Name	Referring Physician	
Smith		Andrea	Fox, Wilson, MD	

Age	Gender	Phone	Exam	
34	F	(478)555-1111	MRI L-Spine Without Contrast	

History

34 y/o female with LBP and numbness in the left lower extremity.

BUN	Creatinine	GFR	
0.00	0.00	0.00	

Notes

GENERAL MEDICAL CENTER
MRI Screening Form

Patient Name: _Andrea Smith_ **Sex:** ☐M ☑F **Weight:** _161_

Age: _34_ **Referring Physician:** _Dr. Wilson Fox_

Please explain the reason for which you are having an MRI exam:
Back pain and numbness in the left leg

Do you have or have you ever had any of the following?

☐ Yes ☑No	Cardiac Pacemaker
☐ Yes ☑No	Heart Surgery/Heart Valve
☐ Yes ☑No	Implanted Cardiac Defibrillator (ICD)
☐ Yes ☑No	Brain Surgery / Brain Aneurysm Clips
☐ Yes ☑No	Shunts/Stents/Filters/Intravascular Coil
☐ Yes ☑No	Eye Surgery/Implants/Spring/Wires/Retinal Tack
☐Yes ☑No	Eye Injury Involving Metal/Metal Shavings
☐Yes ☑No	Orthopedic Pins/Screws/Rods/Joints/Prosthesis
☐Yes ☑No	Neurostimulator / Biostimulator
☐Yes ☑No	Previous Neck/Back Surgery
☐Yes ☑No	Ear Surgery/Cochlear Implants/Hearing Aids
☐Yes ☑No	Vascular Access Port/Catheter
☐Yes ☑No	Metal Implants/Sutures/Staples or Clips
☐Yes ☑No	Electrical/Mechanical/Magnetic Implants
☐Yes ☑No	Implanted Drug Infusion Pump/Insulin Pump
☐Yes ☑No	Are you Pregnant?
☐Yes ☑No	Tattoo's/Permanent Make-up
☑Yes ☐No	Body Piercing, Location _____Ears_____
☐Yes ☑No	Dentures/Partials/Dental Implants
☐Yes ☑No	Gunshot or Shrapnel Wounds
☐Yes ☑No	Do you have pins in your Hair/Clothes?
☐Yes ☑No	Do you have Hair Extensions/Hair Pieces/Wig?
☐Yes ☑No	Do you have any history of kidney disease?
☐Yes ☑No	Do you have any history of hypertension?
☐Yes ☑No	Do you have any history of diabetes?

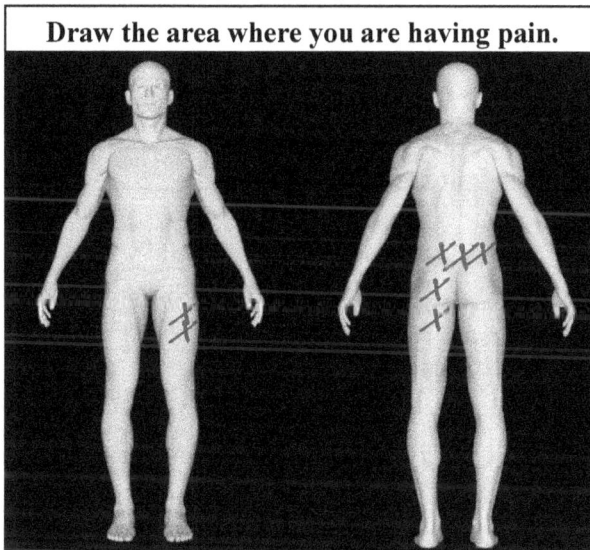

Draw the area where you are having pain.

List Previous Surgeries:
None

I attest that the above information is correct to the best of my knowledge.

X____Andrea Smith_____ _____ _____
Patient/Parent/Legal Guardian **MRI Technologist's Signature** **Date**

Protocol

Protocol: Lumbar Spine Without Contrast

Parameters	Sagittal T1	Sagittal T2	Axial T2	Axial T1
Patient Position	Supine	Supine	Supine	Supine
Patient Entry	Head First	Head First	Head First	Head First
Imaging Coil	CTL Spine Coil	CTL Spine Coil	CTL Spine Coil	CTL Spine Coil
Imaging Plane	Sagittal	Sagittal	Axial	Axial
Pulse Sequence	T1 SE	T2 FSE	T2 FSE	T1 SE
TR	450	3800	5500	400
TE	15	120	100	10
Flip Angle	90	90	90	90
ETL	0	30	12	0
Field of View	28 cm	28 cm	20 cm	20 cm
Slice Thickness	4.0 mm	4.0 mm	4.0 mm	4.0 mm
Slice Spacing	5.0 mm	5.0 mm	5.0 mm	5.0 mm
No. of Slices	12	12	27	27
Start Location	L-19	L-19	S-28	S-28
End Location	R-36	R-36	I - 101	I-101
Freq. Matrix	256	265	256	256
Phase Matrix	256	265	256	256
NSA (Averages)	2	2	2	2
Phase Direction	A/P	A/P	A/P	A/P
Freq. Direction	S/I	S/I	L/R	L/R

Slice Reference

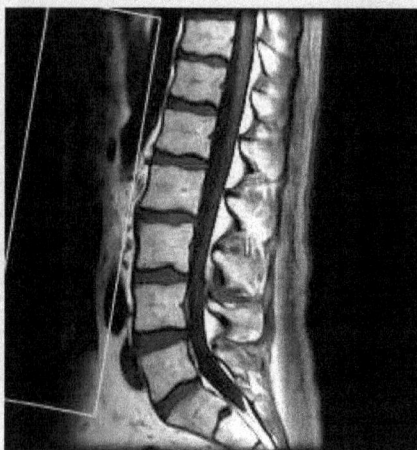

A presaturation pulse can be placed anteriorly in order to suppress flow and respiratory motion.

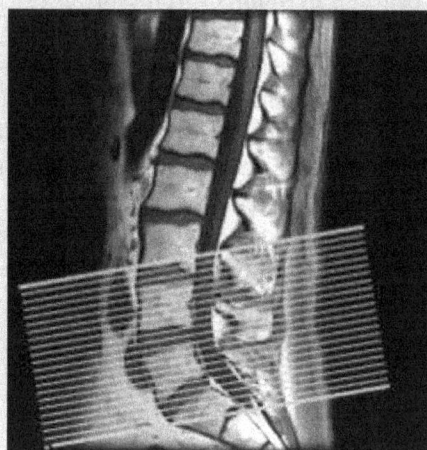

Axial slices should be prescribed so that there is a general angle through the lower 3 disk spaces.

Patient Screening Questions:

1. Is the exam ordered consistent with the patient's history and symptoms? If not, describe why they are not consistent.

_____

_____

_____

_____

_____

_____

_____

_____

2. Are there any contraindications that would prevent the patient from having an MRI exam? If so, list and describe each.

_____

_____

_____

_____

_____

_____

_____

_____

3. Are there any items found on the patient screening form that could cause potential artifacts? If so, please describe .

_____

_____

_____

_____

_____

_____

_____

_____

Exam Performance Questions

4. What type of coil was selected for this procedure?

_____

_____

_____

_____

5. What is the patient's orientation?

_____

_____

_____

_____

6. Were there any artifacts on the images? If so, list the artifact name, list the sequence it appears on, describe its appearance, and define how it should be corrected.

_____

_____

_____

_____

_____

_____

_____

_____

7. Was there any pathology found on the images? If so, list the sequence it appears on and describe its appearance.

_____

_____

_____

_____

_____

_____

_____

_____

8. Describe the two techniques that can be utilized when scanning a lumbar spine to suppress motion artifact from respirations.

_____

_____

_____

_____

_____

_____

_____

_____

_____

9. When would it be important NOT to utilize a saturation pulse to suppress flow artifact from the abdominal aorta?

_____

_____

_____

_____

_____

_____

_____

_____

10. Describe the benefits of utilizing rectangular field of view when scanning the lumbar spine.

_____

_____

_____

_____

_____

_____

_____

_____

NOTES

MRI Lumbar Spine

Objective:

In this lab you will screen the patient, scan an MRI of the lumbar spine without contrast, and evaluate the images.

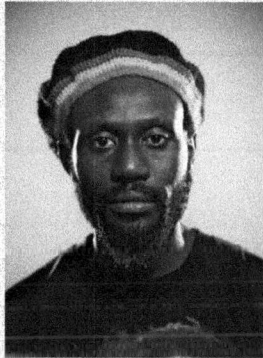

Patient Information

Patient: Wallace, Michael
Age: 41
History: 41 y/o male with Lower back pain and right sided radiculopathy..
Referring Physician: Lisa Jackson, MD

I. PATIENT SCREENING:

A. Evaluate the patient requisition.
B. Evaluate and sign the patient's screening form.
C. Answer the patient screening questions.

II. PERFORM EXAM:

A. If there are no contraindications, enter the patient's name and demographic information into the simulator and continue the exam performance steps. If there are contraindications, please halt the study.
B. Select the appropriate coil.
C. Scan the protocol listed on page 12-4. Upon the completion of each sequence evaluate the images for artifacts and pathology.
D. Answer the procedure questions.

General Medical Center
Patient Requisition

Patient ID			Accession Number	
85742			MR857421250	

Last Name	First Name		Referring Physician	
Wallace	Michael		Jackson, Lisa, MD	

Age	Gender	Phone	Exam
41	M	(478)555-1212	MRI L-Spine Without Contrast

History

41 y/o male with Lower back pain and right sided radiculopathy.

BUN	Creatinine	GFR	
0.00	0.00	0.00	

Notes

GENERAL MEDICAL CENTER
MRI Screening Form

Patient Name: _Michael Wallace_ Sex: ☒M ☐F Weight: _195_

Age: _41_ Referring Physician: _Dr. Lisa Jackson_

Please explain the reason for which you are having an MRI exam:
Back pain right leg pain

Do you have or have you ever had any of the following?

☒Yes ☐No	Cardiac Pacemaker
☐Yes ☒No	Heart Surgery/Heart Valve
☐Yes ☒No	Implanted Cardiac Defibrillator (ICD)
☐Yes ☒No	Brain Surgery / Brain Aneurysm Clips
☐Yes ☒No	Shunts/Stents/Filters/Intravascular Coil
☐Yes ☒No	Eye Surgery/Implants/Spring/Wires/Retinal Tack
☐Yes ☒No	Eye Injury Involving Metal/Metal Shavings
☐Yes ☒No	Orthopedic Pins/Screws/Rods/Joints/Prosthesis
☐Yes ☒No	Neurostimulator / Biostimulator
☐Yes ☒No	Previous Neck/Back Surgery
☐Yes ☒No	Ear Surgery/Cochlear Implants/Hearing Aids
☐Yes ☒No	Vascular Access Port/Catheter
☐Yes ☒No	Metal Implants/Sutures/Staples or Clips
☐Yes ☒No	Electrical/Mechanical/Magnetic Implants
☐Yes ☒No	Implanted Drug Infusion Pump/Insulin Pump
☐Yes ☒No	Are you Pregnant?
☐Yes ☒No	Tattoo's/Permanent Make-up
☐Yes ☒No	Body Piercing, Location _____
☐Yes ☒No	Dentures/Partials/Dental Implants
☐Yes ☒No	Gunshot or Shrapnel Wounds
☐Yes ☒No	Do you have pins in your Hair/Clothes?
☐Yes ☒No	Do you have Hair Extensions/Hair Pieces/Wig?
☐Yes ☒No	Do you have any history of kidney disease?
☐Yes ☒No	Do you have any history of hypertension?
☐Yes ☒No	Do you have any history of diabetes?

Draw the area where you are having pain.

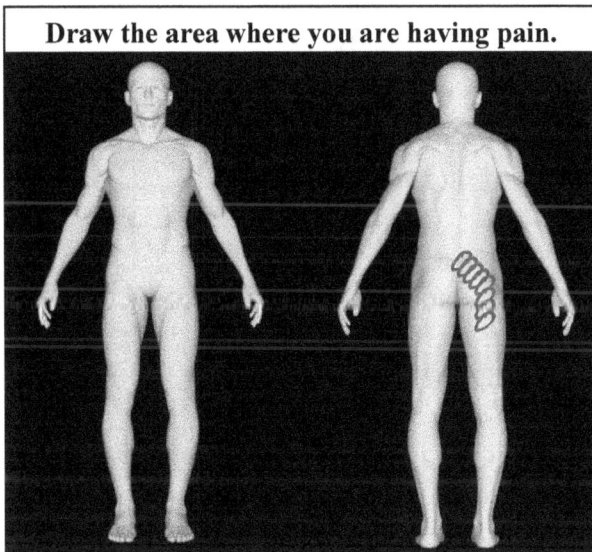

List Previous Surgeries:

Pacemaker Surgery

I attest that the above information is correct to the best of my knowledge.

X_____Michael Wallace_____ _____ _____
Patient/Parent/Legal Guardian MRI Technologist's Signature Date

Protocol

Protocol: Lumbar Spine Without Contrast

Parameters	Sagittal T1	Sagittal T2	Axial T2	Axial T1
Patient Position	Supine	Supine	Supine	Supine
Patient Entry	Head First	Head First	Head First	Head First
Imaging Coil	CTL Spine Coil	CTL Spine Coil	CTL Spine Coil	CTL Spine Coil
Imaging Plane	Sagittal	Sagittal	Axial	Axial
Pulse Sequence	T1 SE	T2 FSE	T2 FSE	T1 SE
TR	450	3800	5500	400
TE	15	120	100	10
Flip Angle	90	90	90	90
ETL	0	30	12	0
Field of View	28 cm	28 cm	20 cm	20 cm
Slice Thickness	4.0 mm	4.0 mm	4.0 mm	4.0 mm
Slice Spacing	5.0 mm	5.0 mm	5.0 mm	5.0 mm
Number of Slices	12	12	27	27
Start Location	L-19	L-19	S-28	S-28
End Location	R-36	R-36	I - 101	I-101
Freq. Matrix	256	265	256	256
Phase Matrix	256	265	256	256
NSA (Averages)	2	2	2	2
Phase Direction	A/P	A/P	A/P	A/P
Freq. Direction	S/I	S/I	L/R	L/R

Slice Reference

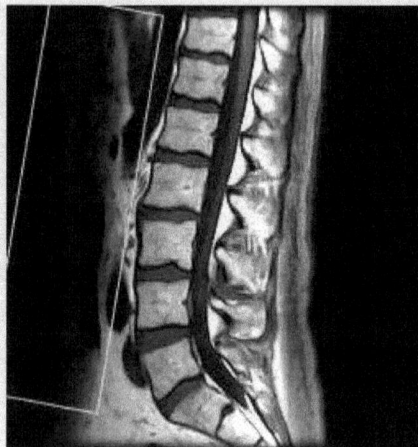

A presaturation pulse can be placed anteriorly in order to suppress flow and respiratory motion.

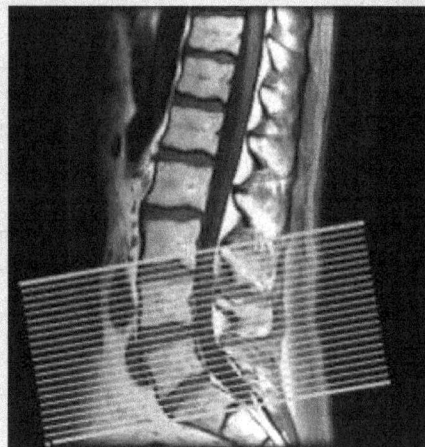

Axial slices should be prescribed so that there is a general angle through the lower 3 disk spaces.

Patient Screening Questions:

1. Is the exam ordered consistent with the patient's history and symptoms? If not, describe why they are not consistent.

_____

_____

_____

_____

_____

_____

_____

_____

2. Are there any contraindications that would prevent the patient from having an MRI exam? If so, list and describe each.

_____

_____

_____

_____

_____

_____

_____

_____

3. Are there any items found on the patient screening form that could cause potential artifacts? If so, please describe.

_____

_____

_____

_____

_____

_____

_____

_____

Exam Performance Questions

4. When scanning a lumbar spine, which patient orientation is most effective for minimizing the effects of claustrophobia?

_____

_____

_____

_____

5. What is the anatomical landmark utilized to position the patient for an MRI of the lumbar spine?

_____

_____

_____

_____

6. Were there any artifacts on the images? If so, list the artifact name, list the sequence it appears on, describe its appearance, and define how it should be corrected.

_____

_____

_____

_____

_____

_____

_____

_____

7. Was there any pathology found on the images? If so, list the sequence it appears on and describe its appearance.

_____

_____

_____

_____

_____

_____

_____

_____

8. Describe the benefits of utilizing a foam pad to elevate the knees when scanning an MRI of the lumbar spine.

_____

_____

_____

_____

_____

_____

_____

_____

NOTES

MRI Lumbar Spine With Contrast

Objective:

In this lab you will screen the patient, scan an MRI of the lumbar spine with contrast, and evaluate the images.

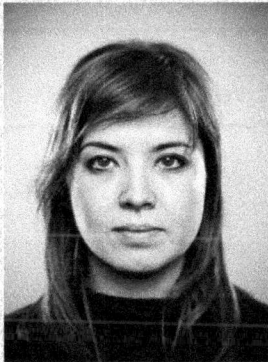

Patient Information

Patient: Andrews, Carolyn
Age: 33
History: 33 y/o female with right lower extremity radiculopathy. Patient has history of previous lumbar surgery
Referring Physician: Robinson, Emory, MD

I. PATIENT SCREENING:

    A. Evaluate the patient requisition.
    B. Evaluate and sign the patient's screening form.
    C. Answer the patient screening questions.
    D. See reference I, II, and VI for the department contrast policy.

II. PERFORM EXAM:

    A. If there are no contraindications, enter the patient's name and demographic information into the simulator and continue the exam performance steps. If there are contraindications, please halt the study.
    B. Select the appropriate coil.
    C. Scan the protocol listed on page 13-4. Upon the completion of each sequence evaluate the images for artifacts and pathology.
    D. Answer the procedure questions.

General Medical Center
Patient Requisition

Patient ID			Accession Number	
95371			MR953713536	

Last Name		First Name	Referring Physician	
Andrews		Carolyn	Robinson, Emory, MD	

Age	Gender	Phone	Exam
33	F	(478)555-1313	MRI L-Spine With Contrast

History

33 y/o female with right lower extremity radiculopathy. Patient has history of previous lumbar surgery.

BUN	Creatinine	GFR	
7.0 mg/dL	1.0 mg/dL	110 mL/min	

Notes

GENERAL MEDICAL CENTER
MRI Screening Form

Patient Name: _Carolyn Andrews_   **Sex:** ☐M ☑F   **Weight:** _115_

Age: _33_   **Referring Physician:** _Dr. Emory Robinson_

Please explain the reason for which you are having an MRI exam:
Weakness in the right leg

Do you have or have you ever had any of the following?

☐ Yes ☑No   Cardiac Pacemaker
☐ Yes ☑No   Heart Surgery/Heart Valve
☐ Yes ☑No   Implanted Cardiac Defibrillator (ICD)
☐ Yes ☑No   Brain Surgery / Brain Aneurysm Clips
☐ Yes ☑No   Shunts/Stents/Filters/Intravascular Coil
☐ Yes ☑No   Eye Surgery/Implants/Spring/Wires/Retinal Tack
☐ Yes ☑No   Eye Injury Involving Metal/Metal Shavings
☐ Yes ☑No   Orthopedic Pins/Screws/Rods/Joints/Prosthesis
☐ Yes ☑No   Neurostimulator / Biostimulator
☑Yes ☐No   Previous Neck/Back Surgery
☐ Yes ☑No   Ear Surgery/Cochlear Implants/Hearing Aids
☐ Yes ☑No   Vascular Access Port/Catheter
☐ Yes ☑No   Metal Implants/Sutures/Staples or Clips
☐ Yes ☑No   Electrical/Mechanical/Magnetic Implants
☐ Yes ☑No   Implanted Drug Infusion Pump/Insulin Pump
☐ Yes ☑No   Are you Pregnant?
☐ Yes ☑No   Tattoo's/Permanent Make-up
☑Yes ☐No   Body Piercing, Location ___Ears___
☐ Yes ☑No   Dentures/Partials/Dental Implants
☐ Yes ☑No   Gunshot or Shrapnel Wounds
☐ Yes ☑No   Do you have pins in your Hair/Clothes?
☐ Yes ☑No   Do you have Hair Extensions/Hair Pieces/Wig?

☐ Yes ☑No   Do you have any history of kidney disease?
☐ Yes ☑No   Do you have any history of hypertension?
☐ Yes ☑No   Do you have any history of diabetes?

Draw the area where you are having pain.

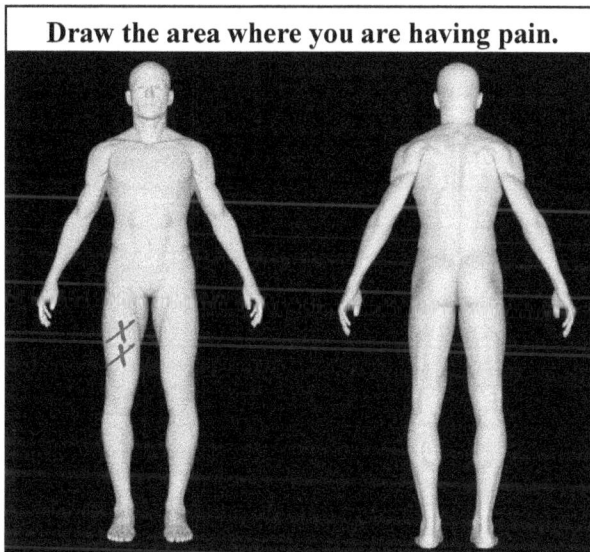

List Previous Surgeries:
Lower back surgery

I attest that the above information is correct to the best of my knowledge.

X___Carolyn Andrews___   _____   _____
Patient/Parent/Legal Guardian   **MRI Technologist's Signature**   **Date**

Protocol

Protocol: Lumbar Spine With Contrast

Parameters	Sagittal T1	Sagittal T2	Axial T2	Axial T1	Axial T1 Post	Sagittal T1 Post
Patient Position	Supine	Supine	Supine	Supine	Supine	Supine
Patient Entry	Head First	Head First	Head First	Head First	Head First	Head First
Imaging Coil	CTL Spine	CTL Spine	CTL Spine	CTL Spine	CTL Spine	CTL Spine
Imaging Plane	Sagittal	Sagittal	Axial	Axial	Axial	Sagittal
Pulse Sequence	T1 SE	T2 FSE	T2 FSE	T1 SE	T1 SE	T1 SE
TR	450	3800	5500	400	400	450
TE	15	120	100	10	10	15
Flip Angle	90	90	90	90	90	90
Echo Train Length	0	30	12	0	0	0
Field of View	28 cm	28 cm	20 cm	20 cm	20 cm	28 cm
Slice Thickness	4.0 mm	4.0 mm	4.0 mm	4.0 mm	4.0 mm	4.0 mm
Slice Spacing	5.0 mm	5.0 mm	5.0 mm	5.0 mm	5.0 mm	5.0 mm
Number of Slices	12	12	27	27	27	12
Start Location	L-19	L-19	S-28	S-28	S-28	L-19
End Location	R-36	R-36	I - 101	I-101	I-101	R-36
Freq. Matrix	256	265	256	256	256	256
Phase Matrix	256	265	256	256	256	256
NSA (Averages)	2	2	2	2	2	2
Phase Direction	A/P	A/P	A/P	A/P	A/P	A/P
Freq. Direction	S/I	S/I	L/R	L/R	L/R	S/I

Slice Reference

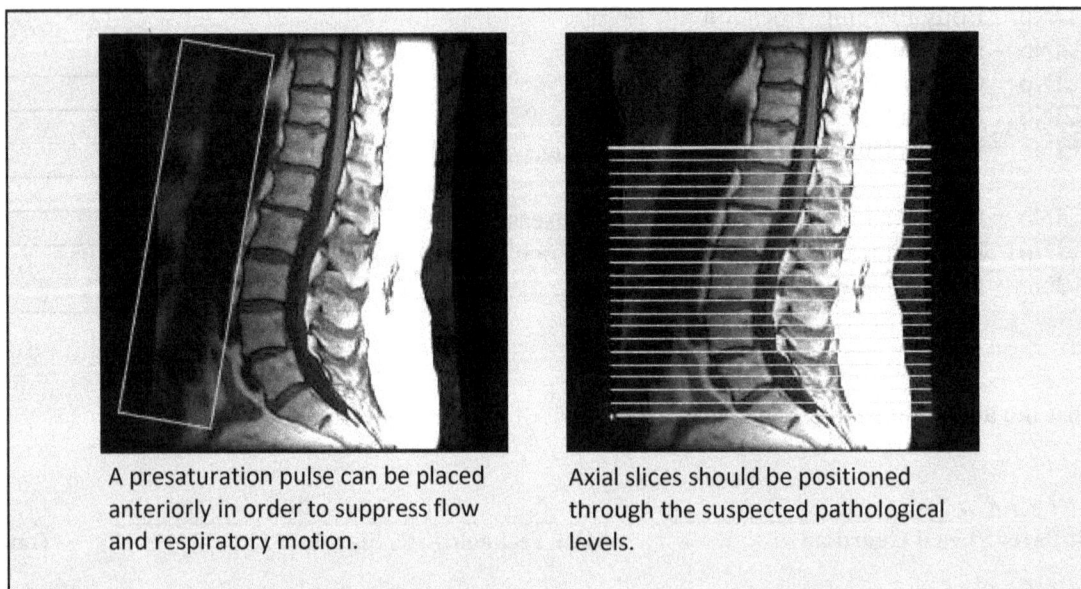

A presaturation pulse can be placed anteriorly in order to suppress flow and respiratory motion.

Axial slices should be positioned through the suspected pathological levels.

Patient Screening Questions:

1. Is the exam ordered consistent with the patient's history and symptoms? If not, describe why they are not consistent.

_____

_____

_____

_____

_____

_____

_____

_____

2. Are there any contraindications that would prevent the patient from having an MRI exam? If so, list and describe each.

_____

_____

_____

_____

_____

_____

_____

_____

_____

3. Are there any items found on the patient screening form that could cause potential artifacts? If so, please describe.

_____

_____

_____

_____

_____

_____

_____

_____

Exam Performance Questions

4. Utilizing the reference chart in the reference section of this book and the patient's weight, calculate the amount of contrast media that should be given.

_____

_____

_____

_____

_____

_____

_____

_____

5. Were there any artifacts on the images? If so, list the artifact name, list the sequence it appears on, describe its appearance, and define how it should be corrected.

_____

_____

_____

_____

_____

_____

_____

_____

6. Was there any pathology found on the images? If so, list the sequence it appears on and describe its appearance.

_____

_____

_____

_____

_____

_____

_____

_____

7. Describe why it is important to utilize gadolinium based contrast media when the patient has had a history of surgery on their lumbar spine.

_____

_____

_____

_____

_____

_____

_____

_____

_____

8. Describe how NSA (Number of Signal Averages) affects the signal to noise ratio and scan time.

_____

_____

_____

_____

_____

_____

_____

_____

_____

NOTES

MRI Shoulder

Objective:

In this lab you will screen the patient, scan an MRI of the shoulder and evaluate the images.

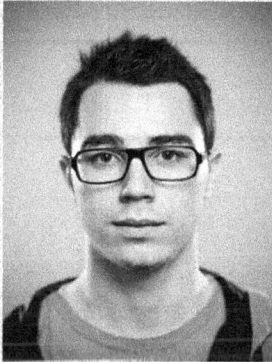

Patient Information

Patient: Daniels, Henry
Age: 17
History: 17 y/o male, r/o right suprascapular nerve entrapment
Referring Physician: Curtis Williams, MD

I. PATIENT SCREENING:

A. Evaluate the patient requisition.
B. Evaluate and sign the patient's screening form.
C. Answer the patient screening questions.

II. PERFORM EXAM:

A. If there are no contraindications, enter the patient's name and demographic information into the simulator and continue the exam performance steps. If there are contraindications, please halt the study.
B. Select the appropriate coil.
C. Scan the protocol listed on page 14-4. Upon the completion of each sequence evaluate the images for artifacts and pathology.
D. Answer the procedure questions.

General Medical Center
Patient Requisition

Patient ID		Accession Number	
356003		MR35600343589	

Last Name	First Name	Referring Physician
Daniels	Henry	Williams, Curtis, MD

Age	Gender	Phone	Exam
17	M	(478)555-1414	MRI Right Shoulder

History

17 y/o male, r/o right suprascapular nerve entrapment

BUN	Creatinine	GFR	
0.00	0.00	0.00	

Notes

GENERAL MEDICAL CENTER
MRI Screening Form

Patient Name: _Henry Daniels_ **Sex:** ☑ M ☐ F **Weight:** _145_

Age: _17_ **Referring Physician:** _Dr. Curtis Williams_

Please explain the reason for which you are having an MRI exam:
Right Shoulder Pain

Do you have or have you ever had any of the following?

☐ Yes	☑ No	Cardiac Pacemaker
☐ Yes	☑ No	Heart Surgery/Heart Valve
☐ Yes	☑ No	Implanted Cardiac Defibrillator (ICD)
☐ Yes	☑ No	Brain Surgery / Brain Aneurysm Clips
☐ Yes	☑ No	Shunts/Stents/Filters/Intravascular Coil
☐ Yes	☑ No	Eye Surgery/Implants/Spring/Wires/Retinal Tack
☐ Yes	☑ No	Eye Injury Involving Metal/Metal Shavings
☐ Yes	☑ No	Orthopedic Pins/Screws/Rods/Joints/Prosthesis
☐ Yes	☑ No	Neurostimulator / Biostimulator
☐ Yes	☑ No	Previous Neck/Back Surgery
☐ Yes	☑ No	Ear Surgery/Cochlear Implants/Hearing Aids
☐ Yes	☑ No	Vascular Access Port/Catheter
☐ Yes	☑ No	Metal Implants/Sutures/Staples or Clips
☐ Yes	☑ No	Electrical/Mechanical/Magnetic Implants
☐ Yes	☑ No	Implanted Drug Infusion Pump/Insulin Pump
☐ Yes	☑ No	Are you Pregnant?
☐ Yes	☑ No	Tattoo's/Permanent Make-up
☐ Yes	☑ No	Body Piercing, Location _____
☐ Yes	☑ No	Dentures/Partials/Dental Implants
☐ Yes	☑ No	Gunshot or Shrapnel Wounds
☐ Yes	☑ No	Do you have pins in your Hair/Clothes?
☐ Yes	☑ No	Do you have Hair Extensions/Hair Pieces/Wig?
☐ Yes	☑ No	Do you have any history of kidney disease?
☐ Yes	☑ No	Do you have any history of hypertension?
☐ Yes	☑ No	Do you have any history of diabetes?

Draw the area where you are having pain.

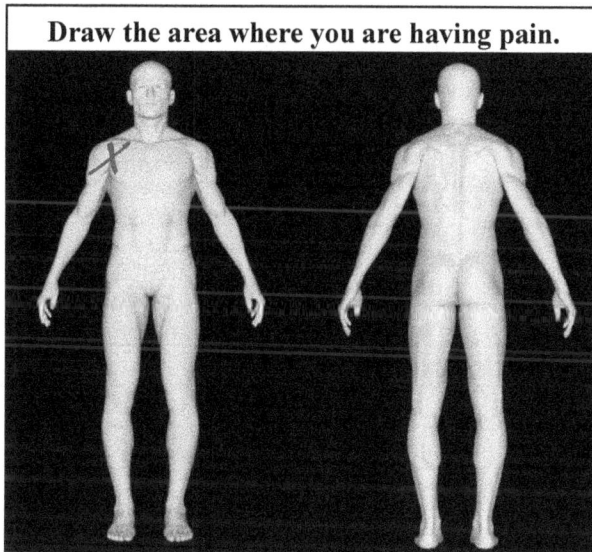

List Previous Surgeries:

None

I attest that the above information is correct to the best of my knowledge.

X_____Henry Daniels_____   _____   _____
Patient/Parent/Legal Guardian   **MRI Technologist's Signature**   **Date**

Protocol

Protocol: Shoulder

Parameters	Scout	Axial T1	Coronal T1	Coronal T2	Sagittal T1
Patient Position	Supine	Supine	Supine	Supine	Supine
Patient Entry	Head First	Head First	Head First	Head First	Head First
Imaging Coil	Shoulder	Shoulder	Shoulder	Shoulder	Shoulder
Imaging Plane	MP	Axial	Coronal	Coronal	Sagittal
Pulse Sequence	T2 GRE	T1 SE	T1 SE	T2 FSE	T1 SE
TR	65	550	600	2000	420
TE	2	22	14	70	14
Flip Angle	30	90	90	90	90
ETL	0	0	0	6	0
Field of View	24 cm	14 cm	14 cm	14 cm	14 cm
Slice Thickness	5.0 mm	4.0 mm	4.0 mm	4.0 mm	4.0 mm
Slice Spacing	7.0 mm	4.0 mm	4.0 mm	4.0 mm	4.0 mm
Number of Slices	21	14	16	16	22
Start Location	X	S-40	A-54	A-54	R-212
End Location	X	I-12	A-10	A-10	R-150
Freq. Matrix	256	256	256	256	256
Phase Matrix	256	256	256	256	256
NSA (Averages)	1	2	2	2	2
Phase Direction	A/P	A/P	L/R	L/R	A/P
Freq. Direction	S/I	L/R	S/I	L/R	S/I

Slice Reference

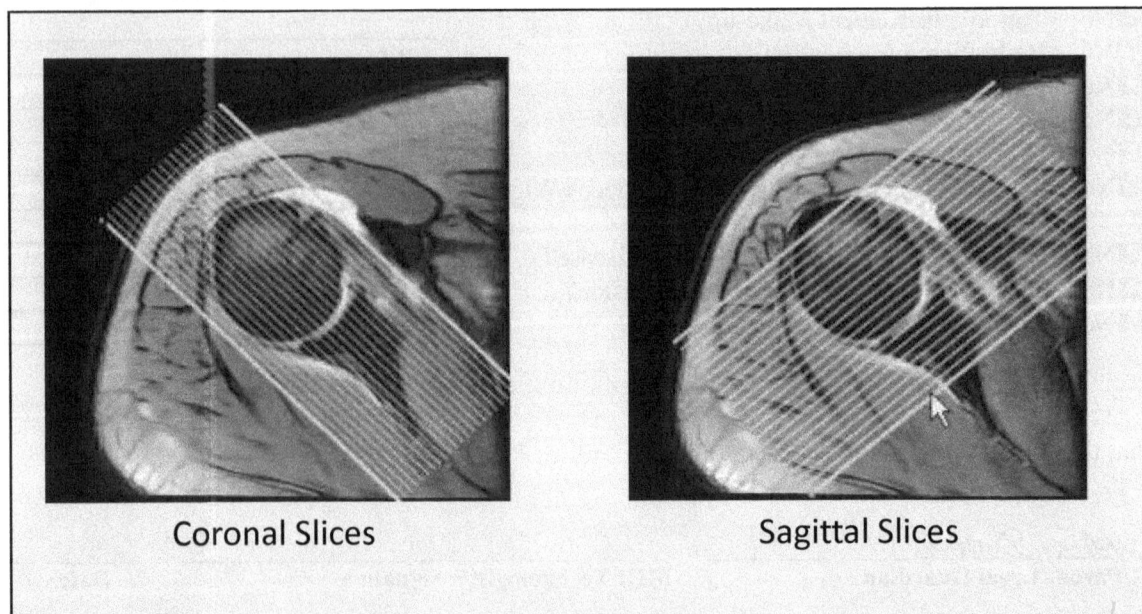

Coronal Slices

Sagittal Slices

Patient Screening Questions:

1. Is the exam ordered consistent with the patient's history and symptoms? If not, describe why they are not consistent.

_____

_____

_____

_____

_____

_____

_____

_____

2. Are there any contraindications that would prevent the patient from having an MRI exam? If so, list and describe each.

_____

_____

_____

_____

_____

_____

_____

_____

_____

3. Are there any items found on the patient screening form that could cause potential artifacts? If so, please describe .

_____

_____

_____

_____

_____

_____

_____

_____

Exam Performance Questions

4. What type of coil was selected for this procedure?

_____
_____
_____
_____

5. What is the patient's orientation?

_____
_____
_____
_____

6. Were there any artifacts on the images? If so, list the artifact name, list the sequence it appears on, describe its appearance, and define how it should be corrected.

_____
_____
_____
_____
_____
_____
_____
_____

7. Was there any pathology found on the images? If so, list the sequence it appears on and describe its appearance.

_____
_____
_____
_____
_____
_____
_____
_____

8. When setting up a coronal sequence of the shoulder from an axial scout, slices should be prescribed parallel to which muscle?

_____

_____

_____

_____

_____

_____

_____

_____

_____

9. Describe how the patient's arm should be positioned when scanning the shoulder.

_____

_____

_____

_____

_____

_____

_____

_____

_____

10. Describe "magic angle" artifact and how it can be minimized when scanning the shoulder.

_____

_____

_____

_____

_____

_____

_____

_____

_____

NOTES

MRI Knee

Objective:

In this lab you will screen the patient, scan an MRI of the knee, and evaluate the images.

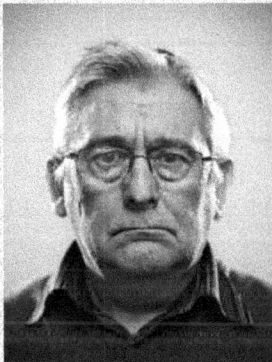

Patient Information

Patient: Wilson, Forrest
Age: 65
History: 65 y/o male with injury to the knee during a fall.
Referring Physician: Emily Walker, MD

I. PATIENT SCREENING:

A. Evaluate the patient requisition.
B. Evaluate and sign the patient's screening form.
C. Answer the patient screening questions.
D. See lab reference V for Lab 15.

II. PERFORM EXAM:

A. If there are no contraindications, enter the patient's name and demographic information into the simulator and continue the exam performance steps. If there are contraindications, please halt the study.
B. Select the appropriate coil.
C. Scan the protocol listed on page 15-4 and 15-5. Upon the completion of each sequence evaluate the images for artifacts and pathology.
D. Answer the procedure questions.

General Medical Center
Patient Requisition

Patient ID	Accession Number
88576	MR88576140

Last Name	First Name	Referring Physician
Wilson	Forrest	Walker, Emily MD

Age	Gender	Phone	Exam
65	M	(478)555-1414	MRI Right Knee

History

65 y/o male with injury to the knee during a fall.

BUN	Creatinine	GFR	
0.00	0.00	0.00	

Notes

GENERAL MEDICAL CENTER
MRI Screening Form

Patient Name: _Forrest Wilson_   Sex: ☒ M ☐ F   Weight: _175_

Age: _65_   Referring Physician: _Dr. Emily Walker_

Please explain the reason for which you are having an MRI exam:
Fell on right knee

Do you have or have you ever had any of the following?

☐ Yes	☒ No	Cardiac Pacemaker
☐ Yes	☒ No	Heart Surgery/Heart Valve
☐ Yes	☒ No	Implanted Cardiac Defibrillator (ICD)
☐ Yes	☒ No	Brain Surgery / Brain Aneurysm Clips
☐ Yes	☒ No	Shunts/Stents/Filters/Intravascular Coil
☐ Yes	☒ No	Eye Surgery/Implants/Spring/Wires/Retinal Tack
☒ Yes	☐ No	Eye Injury Involving Metal/Metal Shavings
☐ Yes	☒ No	Orthopedic Pins/Screws/Rods/Joints/Prosthesis
☐ Yes	☒ No	Neurostimulator / Biostimulator
☐ Yes	☒ No	Previous Neck/Back Surgery
☐ Yes	☒ No	Ear Surgery/Cochlear Implants/Hearing Aids
☐ Yes	☒ No	Vascular Access Port/Catheter
☐ Yes	☒ No	Metal Implants/Sutures/Staples or Clips
☐ Yes	☒ No	Electrical/Mechanical/Magnetic Implants
☐ Yes	☒ No	Implanted Drug Infusion Pump/Insulin Pump
☐ Yes	☒ No	Are you Pregnant?
☐ Yes	☒ No	Tattoo's/Permanent Make-up
☐ Yes	☒ No	Body Piercing, Location _____
☐ Yes	☒ No	Dentures/Partials/Dental Implants
☐ Yes	☒ No	Gunshot or Shrapnel Wounds
☐ Yes	☒ No	Do you have pins in your Hair/Clothes?
☐ Yes	☒ No	Do you have Hair Extensions/Hair Pieces/Wig?
☐ Yes	☒ No	Do you have any history of kidney disease?
☐ Yes	☒ No	Do you have any history of hypertension?
☐ Yes	☒ No	Do you have any history of diabetes?

Draw the area where you are having pain.

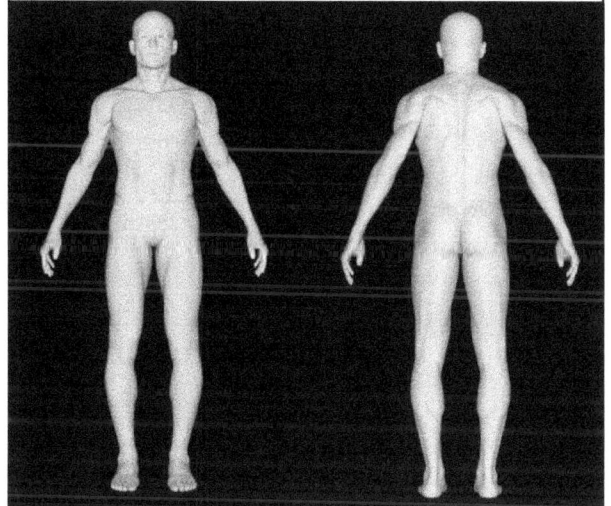

List Previous Surgeries:

None

I attest that the above information is correct to the best of my knowledge.

X____Forrest Wilson_____   _____   _____
Patient/Parent/Legal Guardian   **MRI Technologist's Signature**   **Date**

Protocol (Page 1 of 2)

Protocol: Knee

Parameters	Scout	Coronal T1	Coronal T2	Axial PD
Patient Position	Supine	Supine	Supine	Supine
Patient Entry	Feet First	Feet First	Feet First	Feet First
Imaging Coil	Knee Coil	Knee Coil	Knee Coil	Knee Coil
Imaging Plane	MP	Coronal	Coronal	Axial
Pulse Sequence	T2 GRE	T1 SE	T2 FSE	PD FSE/FS
TR	80	550	4600	3000
TE	2	10	90	25
Flip Angle	30	90	90	90
ETL	0	0	16	8
Field of View	28 cm	16 cm	16 cm	16 cm
Slice Thickness	5.0 mm	4.0 mm	4.0 mm	4.0 mm
Slice Spacing	10.0 mm	5.0 mm	5.0 mm	5.0 mm
No. of Slices	27	20	20	20
Start Location	X	P-46	P-46	I-63
End Location	X	A-44	A-44	S-30
Contrast Amount	0	0	0	0
Contrast Agent	0	0	0	0
Freq. Matrix	256	256	265	256
Phase Matrix	256	256	265	256
NSA (Averages)	1	2	2	2
Phase Direction	L/R	L/R	L/R	L/R
Freq. Direction	A/P	S/I	S/I	A/P

Slice Reference

Axial Slices

Coronal Slices

Sagittal Slices
To best visualize the ACL, the knee should be rotated externally 10° **OR** slices should be rotated 10° internally

Protocol (Page 2 of 2)

Protocol: Knee

Parameters	Axial T2	Sagittal PD	Coronal PD	Sagittal PD	Sagittal T2
Patient Position	Supine	Supine	Supine	Supine	Supine
Patient Entry	Feet First	Feet First	Feet First	Feet First	Feet First
Imaging Coil	Knee Coil	Knee Coil	Knee Coil	Knee Coil	Knee Coil
Imaging Plane	Axial	Sagittal	Coronal	Sagittal	Sagittal
Pulse Sequence	T2 FSE/FS	PD FSE/FS	PD FSE	PD FSE	T2 FSE
TR	3000	3200	2450	3200	2350
TE	90	25	25	25	90
Flip Angle	90	90	90	90	90
ETL	8	8	6	8	0
Field of View	16 cm	18 cm	16 cm	18 cm	16 cm
Slice Thickness	4.0 mm	4.0 mm	4.0 mm	4.0 mm	4.0 mm
Slice Spacing	5.0 mm	5.0 mm	5.0 mm	5.0 mm	5.0 mm
No of Slices	20	21	22	21	21
Start Location	I-63	R-104	P-54	R-104	R-104
End Location	S-30	R-4	A-45	R-4	R-4
Freq. Matrix	256	256	256	256	256
Phase Matrix	256	256	256	256	256
NSA (Averages)	2	2	2	2	1
Phase Direction	L/R	A/P	L/R	A/P	A/P
Freq. Direction	A/P	S/I	S/I	S/I	S/I

Patient Screening Questions:

1. Is the exam ordered consistent with the patient's history and symptoms? If not, describe why they are not consistent.

_____

_____

_____

_____

_____

_____

_____

_____

2. Are there any contraindications that would prevent the patient from having an MRI exam? If so, list and describe each.

_____

_____

_____

_____

_____

_____

_____

_____

3. Are there any items found on the patient screening form that could cause potential artifacts? If so, please describe.

_____

_____

_____

_____

_____

_____

_____

_____

Exam Performance Questions

4. Were there any artifacts on the images? If so, list the artifact name, list the sequence it appears on, describe its appearance, and define how it should be corrected.

_____

_____

_____

_____

_____

_____

_____

_____

_____

_____

5. Was there any pathology found on the images? If so, list the sequence it appears on and describe its appearance.

_____

_____

_____

_____

_____

_____

_____

_____

_____

_____

6. Describe the process that should be used to screen the orbits of patients with potential metallic foreign bodies.

_____

_____

_____

_____

_____

_____

_____

_____

_____

_____

_____

NOTES

MRI Knee

Objective:

In this lab you will screen the patient, scan an MRI of the knee, and evaluate the images.

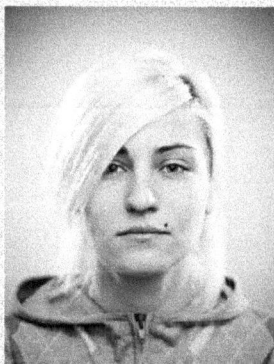

Patient Information

Patient: White, Leslie

Age: 19

History: 19 y/o female with pain and swelling in knee x 3 weeks

Referring Physician: Charles Thomas, MD

I. PATIENT SCREENING:

A. Evaluate the patient requisition.

B. Evaluate and sign the patient's screening form.

C. Answer the patient screening questions.

II. PERFORM EXAM:

A. If there are no contraindications, enter the patient's name and demographic information into the simulator and continue the exam performance steps. If there are contraindications, please halt the study.

B. Select the appropriate coil.

C. Scan the protocol listed on pages 16-4 and 16-5. Upon the completion of each sequence evaluate the images for artifacts and pathology.

D. Answer the procedure questions.

General Medical Center Patient Requisition	
Patient ID 82641	**Accession Number** MR82641353

Last Name White	First Name Leslie	Referring Physician Thomas, Charles MD

Age 19	Gender F	Phone (478)555-1616	Exam MRI Right Knee

History

19 y/o female with pain and swelling in knee x 3 weeks

BUN 0.00	Creatinine 0.00	GFR 0.00	

Notes

GENERAL MEDICAL CENTER
MRI Screening Form

Patient Name: _Leslie White_   Sex: ☐M ☒F   Weight: _132_

Age: _19_   Referring Physician: _Dr. Charles Thomas_

Please explain the reason for which you are having an MRI exam:
Right knee pain and swelling

Do you have or have you ever had any of the following?

☐ Yes	☒ No	Cardiac Pacemaker
☐ Yes	☒ No	Heart Surgery/Heart Valve
☐ Yes	☒ No	Implanted Cardiac Defibrillator (ICD)
☐ Yes	☒ No	Brain Surgery / Brain Aneurysm Clips
☐ Yes	☒ No	Shunts/Stents/Filters/Intravascular Coil
☐ Yes	☒ No	Eye Surgery/Implants/Spring/Wires/Retinal Tack
☐ Yes	☒ No	Eye Injury Involving Metal/Metal Shavings
☐ Yes	☒ No	Orthopedic Pins/Screws/Rods/Joints/Prosthesis
☐ Yes	☒ No	Neurostimulator / Biostimulator
☐ Yes	☒ No	Previous Neck/Back Surgery
☐ Yes	☒ No	Ear Surgery/Cochlear Implants/Hearing Aids
☐ Yes	☒ No	Vascular Access Port/Catheter
☐ Yes	☒ No	Metal Implants/Sutures/Staples or Clips
☐ Yes	☒ No	Electrical/Mechanical/Magnetic Implants
☐ Yes	☒ No	Implanted Drug Infusion Pump/Insulin Pump
☐ Yes	☒ No	Are you Pregnant?
☐ Yes	☒ No	Tattoo's/Permanent Make-up
☒ Yes	☐ No	Body Piercing, Location _Ears, Lip_
☐ Yes	☒ No	Dentures/Partials/Dental Implants
☐ Yes	☒ No	Gunshot or Shrapnel Wounds
☐ Yes	☒ No	Do you have pins in your Hair/Clothes?
☐ Yes	☒ No	Do you have Hair Extensions/Hair Pieces/Wig?
☐ Yes	☒ No	Do you have any history of kidney disease?
☐ Yes	☒ No	Do you have any history of hypertension?
☐ Yes	☒ No	Do you have any history of diabetes?

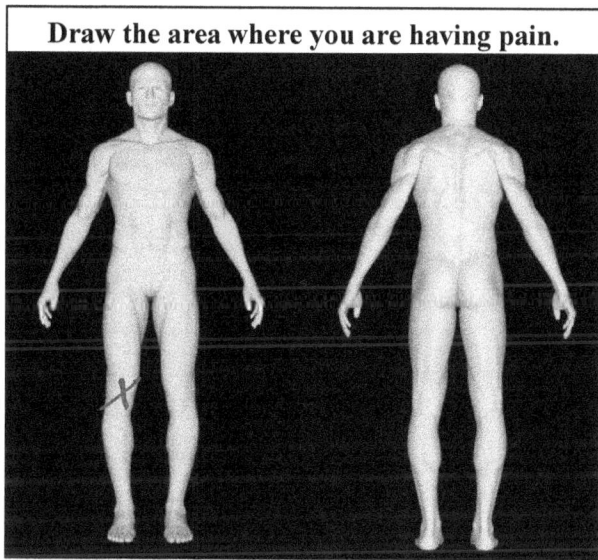

Draw the area where you are having pain.

List Previous Surgeries:
None

I attest that the above information is correct to the best of my knowledge.

X _Leslie White_

Patient/Parent/Legal Guardian   **MRI Technologist's Signature**   **Date**

Protocol (Page 1 of 2)

Protocol: Knee

Parameters	Scout	Coronal T1	Coronal T2	Axial PD
Patient Position	Supine	Supine	Supine	Supine
Patient Entry	Feet First	Feet First	Feet First	Feet First
Imaging Coil	Knee Coil	Knee Coil	Knee Coil	Knee Coil
Imaging Plane	MP	Coronal	Coronal	Axial
Pulse Sequence	T2 GRE	T1 SE	T2 FSE	PD FSE/FS
TR	80	550	4600	3000
TE	2	10	90	25
Flip Angle	30	90	90	90
ETL	0	0	16	8
Field of View	28 cm	16 cm	16 cm	16 cm
Slice Thickness	5.0 mm	4.0 mm	4.0 mm	4.0 mm
Slice Spacing	10.0 mm	5.0 mm	5.0 mm	5.0 mm
Number of Slices	27	20	20	20
Start Location	X	P-46	P-46	I-63
End Location	X	A-44	A-44	S-30
Contrast Amount	0	0	0	0
Contrast Agent	0	0	0	0
Freq. Matrix	256	256	265	256
Phase Matrix	256	256	265	256
NSA (Averages)	1	2	2	2
Phase Direction	L/R	L/R	L/R	L/R
Freq. Direction	A/P	S/I	S/I	A/P

Slice Reference

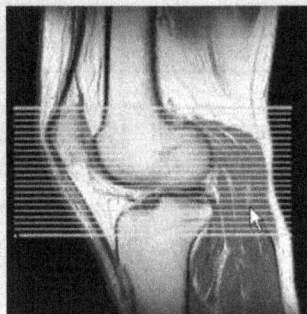

Axial Slices

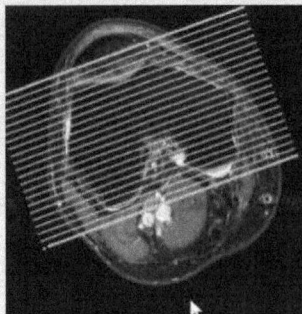

Coronal Slices

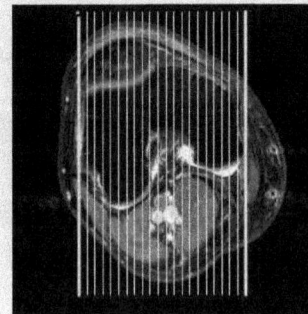

Sagittal Slices
To best visualize the ACL, the knee should be rotated externally 10° **OR** slices should be rotated 10° internally

---

Protocol (Page 2 of 2)

Protocol: Knee

Parameters	Axial T2	Sagittal PD	Coronal PD	Sagittal PD	Sagittal T2
Patient Position	Supine	Supine	Supine	Supine	Supine
Patient Entry	Feet First	Feet First	Feet First	Feet First	Feet First
Imaging Coil	Knee Coil	Knee Coil	Knee Coil	Knee Coil	Knee Coil
Imaging Plane	Axial	Sagittal	Coronal	Sagittal	Sagittal
Pulse Sequence	T2 FSE/FS	PD FSE/FS	PD FSE	PD FSE	T2 FSE
TR	3000	3200	2450	3200	2350
TE	90	25	25	25	90
Flip Angle	90	90	90	90	90
ETL	8	8	6	8	0
Field of View	16 cm	18 cm	16 cm	18 cm	16 cm
Slice Thickness	4.0 mm	4.0 mm	4.0 mm	4.0 mm	4.0 mm
Slice Spacing	5.0 mm	5.0 mm	5.0 mm	5.0 mm	5.0 mm
Number of Slices	20	21	22	21	21
Start Location	I-63	R-104	P-54	R-104	R-104
End Location	S-30	R-4	A- 45	R-4	R-4
Freq. Matrix	256	256	256	256	256
Phase Matrix	256	256	256	256	256
NSA (Averages)	2	2	2	2	1
Phase Direction	L/R	A/P	L/R	A/P	A/P
Freq. Direction	A/P	S/I	S/I	S/I	S/I

Patient Screening Questions:

1. Is the exam ordered consistent with the patient's history and symptoms? If not, describe why they are not consistent.

_____

_____

_____

_____

_____

_____

_____

_____

_____

2. Are there any contraindications that would prevent the patient from having an MRI exam? If so, list and describe each.

_____

_____

_____

_____

_____

_____

_____

_____

_____

3. Are there any items found on the patient screening form that could cause potential artifacts? If so, please describe .

_____

_____

_____

_____

_____

_____

_____

_____

Exam Performance Questions

4. Which anatomical landmark is utilized to position the patient for an MRI of the knee?

_____

_____

_____

_____

_____

_____

_____

_____

5. Were there any artifacts on the images? If so, list the artifact name, list the sequence it appears on, describe its appearance, and define how it should be corrected.

_____

_____

_____

_____

_____

_____

_____

_____

_____

6. Was there any pathology found on the images? If so, list the sequence it appears on and describe its appearance.

_____

_____

_____

_____

_____

_____

_____

_____

_____

7. Describe why its important to angle the slices or rotate the knee approximately 5° to 10° externally when scanning a sagittal sequence of the knee.

_____

_____

_____

_____

_____

_____

_____

_____

8. Describe the common cause of flow artifact on an MRI of the knee and how to minimize its affects on image quality.

_____

_____

_____

_____

_____

_____

_____

_____

NOTES

I. Normal Laboratory Values

Lab Value	Normal Range	
	Men	Women
BUN	7 - 20 mg/dL	7 - 20 mg/dL
Serum Creatinine	0.5 - 1.5 mg/dL	0.6 - 1.2 mg/dL
eGFR	> 90 ml/min/1.72m^2	> 90 ml/min/1.72m^2

II. MRI Intravenous Contrast Policy

Laboratory results should be checked for the most recent serum creatinine/eGFR on ALL patients (by the technologist performing the study).

For patients with the following risk factors, serum creatinine should be performed within 6 weeks of the MRI study:

1. Age 60 years or older
2. Diabetes requiring medication
3. Hypertension requiring medication
4. Kidney disease (including solitary kidney or renal transplant)
5. Family history of kidney disease
6. Organ transplantation
7. Multiple myeloma

For patients with the following risk factors, serum creatinine/eGFR should be performed within 24 hours of the MRI study:

1. Liver failure
2. In-patient or ER patient

eGFR (ml/min/1.72m^2)	IV Gadolinium Based Contrast Use
< 30	Not recommended If gadolinium essential use lowest possible dose with approval of attending radiologist Informed consent must be obtained
30 - 60	Use minimum/ single dose of Multihance
> 60	No restrictions
History of severe renal and/or liver disease	Not recommended If gadolinium essential use lowest possible dose. with approval of attending radiologist Informed consent must be obtained

III. LAB 3 Aneurysm Clip Search Results

The patient did not know what type of aneurysm clip that was used. However, the surgeon's office was contacted and confirmed that the following type of clip was used:

Sundt-Kees Multi-Angle
(17-7PH) aneurysm clip
Downs Surgical, Inc.
Decatur, GA

IV. LAB 7 Orbit Screening and Greenfield Filter Search Results

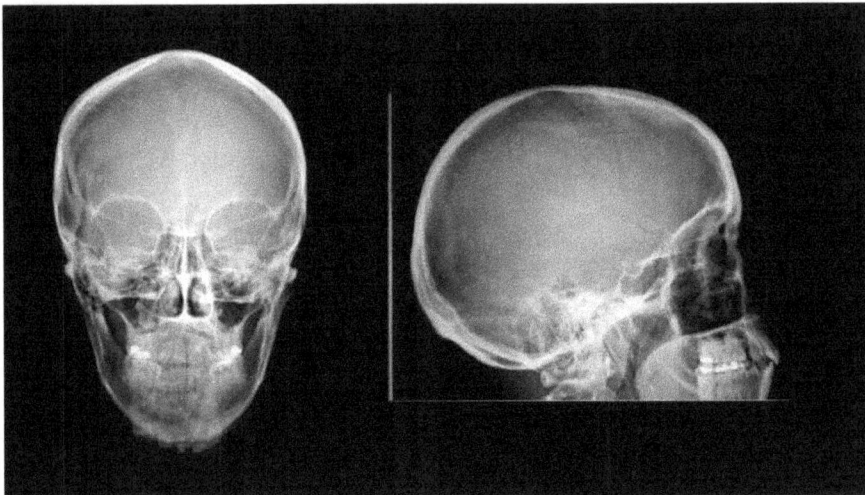

Results: Normal, no metal found in the orbits.

The patient produced a card that included the following information about the Greenfield filter that was used.

Greenfield vena cava filter (titanium alloy)
coil, stent, filter
Ormco
Glendora, CA

V. LAB 15 Orbit Screening Results

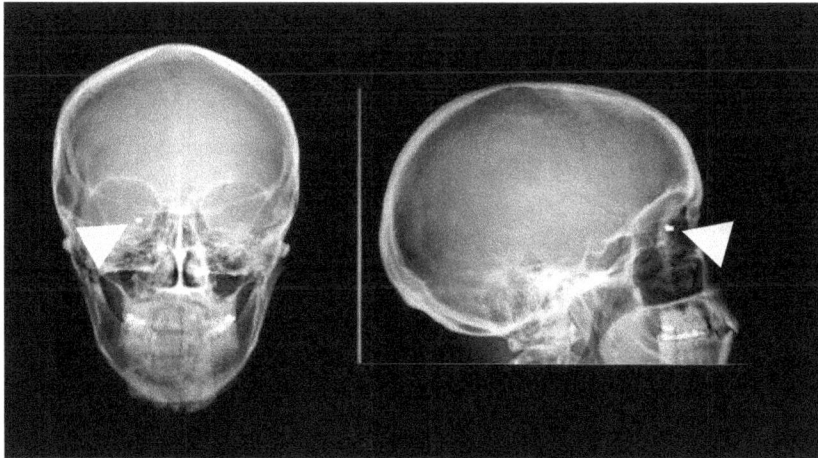

Results: Metal was found in the right orbit. The MRI procedures should not be performed.

VI. LABs Requiring Gadolinium Based Contrast Injections

The recommended dosage of MAGNEVIST Injection is 0.2 mL/kg (0.1 mmol/ kg) administered intravenously, at a rate not to exceed 10 mL per 15 seconds. Dosing for patients in excess of 286 lbs has not been studied systematically.

DOSE AND DURATION OF GADOLINIUM INJECTION BY BODY WEIGHT		
BODY WEIGHT		Total Volume, mL*
lbs	kg	
22	10	2
44	20	4
66	30	6
88	40	8
110	50	10
132	60	12
154	70	14
176	80	16
198	90	18
220	100	20
242	110	22
264	120	24
286	130	26
Rate of Injection:10 mL/15sec	**Rate of Injection:10 mL/15sec	*Rate of Injection:10 mL/15sec

VII. Calculating Scan Time

Conventional Spin Echo: Scan time = TR x NEX x Phase matrix

Fast Spin Echo: Scan time = $\dfrac{\text{TR x NEX x Phase matrix}}{\text{ETL}}$

VIII. Scan Time Conversions

1000 milliseconds = 1 second
1 millisecond = .001 seconds

www.ingramcontent.com/pod-product-compliance
Lightning Source LLC
Chambersburg PA
CBHW082036230326
41598CB00081B/6525